All About

Breast Cancer

FRED STEPHENS

AM MD MS FRCS(Ed) FACS FRACS
Professor Emeritus and former Head,
Department of Surgery,
University of Sydney;
Consultant Emeritus in Surgical Oncology,
Sydney Hospital and Royal Prince Alfred
Hospital, Sydney, Australia

Foreword

I am pleased to recommend this book, and I believe I have a responsibility to support it. I know from personal experience what a mysterious and scary thing it is to receive a life-threatening diagnosis. I know what it's like to need to talk, to want to ask many questions, to have the expert take time to go through all the 'ifs and buts' with me as a person, not as a scientific problem or as a lump of breast tissue with a problem. Unfortunately I also know from personal experience that in some instances doctors do not or cannot always provide the quality time that the cancer sufferer needs.

That's where a book like this is vital—it brings a comforting bedside manner as well as scientific knowledge to the individual. It describes with sensitivity the many different personal responses a woman might have when learning about her disease; you realise you're not alone, and it makes a complicated and frightening experience real and manageable. This book is long overdue, with its unique approach of combining the personal and the scientific in everyday terms. It explains what a breast cancer is, with many grades of seriousness, and simply and clearly explains all the recommended methods of treatment.

I think this is a book for doctors, too. It is written in real everyday language, the kind of language that we everyday people need to hear, to help us understand the problem. It also helps us to appreciate that doctors can be understanding and caring people who can speak with their patients as friends in a way that helps them understand.

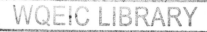

Fred Stephens has a lot of degrees, but he certainly has not taken a degree in aloofness, as some doctors seem to have. He might have taken a very essential degree, one in undertanding and compassion and human relations, traditionally and proudly called by the medical profession a 'bedside manner'.

I highly recommend this book for all those with a breast cancer or who are worried about the disease. I also recommend it to those in the health professions, caring or learning to care for women with breast cancer or indeed any other serious health problem. This book shows how to bridge the gap that can be a barrier between expert and lay person in the communication so essential to good health care.

Raelene Boyle

Dedication

I am pleased to dedicate this book to my wonderful family. As a husband, father, father-in-law, and grandfather it is a constant delight to have such a close and devoted family, every member of which I am very proud of and love dearly.

I am also greatly privileged to have a large, close, and warm extended family of brothers, sisters, in-laws, nieces, nephews, and cousins. They have always been supportive of my work. My late mum and dad, Dorys and Hedley Stephens of the little village of Kurmond, set us all a good example in their love and goodness from which we all benefited.

With this book I especially remember my late sister Heather, who battled this cancer with great courage.

OXFORD

253 Normanby Road, South Melbourne, Victoria, Australia

Oxford University Press is a department of the University of Oxford.
It furthers the University's objective of excellence in research, scholarship,
and education by publishing worldwide in

Oxford New York

Athens Auckland Bangkok Bogotá Buenos Aires
Cape Town Chennai Dar es Salaam Delhi Florence
Hong Kong Istanbul Karachi Kolkata Kuala Lumpur
Madrid Melbourne Mexico City Mumbai Nairobi
Paris Port Moresby São Paulo Shanghai Singapore
Taipei Tokyo Toronto
and associated companies in
Berlin Ibadan

OXFORD is a trade mark of Oxford University Press

National Library of Australia
Cataloguing-in-publication data:

Stephens, Fred.
All about breast cancer.

Bibliography.
Includes index.
ISBN 0 19 551396 7.

1. Breast—Cancer—Popular works. I. Title.

616.99449

Edited by Elaine Cochrane
Indexed by Russell Brooks
Cover designed by Modern Art Production Group
Cover photograph from PhotoDisc
Typeset by Solo Typesetting, South Australia
Printed through Bookpac Production Services, Singapore

Contents

Illustrations

Tables

Acknowledgments

I acknowledge with gratitude considerable help from family and friends, who read earlier manuscripts of this book to ensure that it was written in a style and in language easily understood by patients and people who do not have a medical background. Especially helpful were my wife, Sheilagh, my daughter, Katie, and my friends Lyn Stewart, Valerie Corrigan, Dr John and Mrs Rose Watson. Professor John Boyages, a director of the Australian Cancer Society, kindly read the manuscript and made some very helpful suggestions.

As always Dr John Knight was encouraging and helpful in advising about the scope of this book for patients and doctors in family practice. Dr Paul MacKenzie, Dr Nigel Hunter, and Professor George Ramsay-Stewart kindly supplied illustrations 2.1, 5.4(b) and 5.5 respectively. All members of the Audio-Visual Department of the Royal Prince Alfred Hospital helped beyond their normal duties in preparing the illustrations, and Mr Bob Haynes converted my rough illustrations into meaningful diagrams. Dr David Pennington, head of Plastic and Reconstructive Surgery at the Royal Prince Alfred Hospital, kindly provided the photographs of one of his patients with breast reconstruction (figures 10.1 (a) and (b)).

I acknowledge with thanks much publishing assistance. The ready cooperation and professional editorial help of Elaine Cochrane, and ready and constructive advice and help in publishing and other matters from all members of Oxford University

Press with whom I have had contact, have been much appreciated. Cathryn Game, Heather Fawcett, Ray O'Farrell, and their assistants have always responded to my many enquiries promptly and constructively.

I am especially thankful to Miss Raelene Boyle, who readily agreed to read the manuscript and to write the foreword. In her busy life Raelene always finds time to help charities and especially cancer research charities. We first met at meetings to establish the Sporting Chance Foundation for cancer research. I am pleased to recommend the Sporting Chance Foundation as very worthy of support for its good work. My other strong recommendation for any kind benefactor is that the Chair of Surgical Oncology at the University of Sydney, which I held on a personal basis until I retired, now be established on a permanent basis. Much progress has been made in cancer research and treatment, and it should continue.

Introduction

Breast cancer became increasingly common in women of Western societies during the twentieth century. Other than skin cancer, it is now the most common cancer of women in Western countries, although in some countries lung cancer has become about as common as breast cancer as a consequence of increased smoking rates among women. Breast cancer is less common in Asian, African and most South American countries, especially in their less Westernised and 'less developed' communities. A small number of men in all communities also develop breast cancer.

There are probably many reasons for the difference in incidence. Inherited genetic factors probably play a part, and possibly racial and social factors. The most clearly recognised factor is the age at which women give birth, and whether they breast-feed their babies. In countries where breast cancer is not common, the age at which women give birth to their first child is generally lower than in Western countries, and prolonged breast-feeding of babies is the normal practice.

More recently attention has been given to a possible relationship with diet. There is a distinctly lower incidence of breast cancer in communities where standard diets contain relatively large quantities of plant food. The high content of the natural plant hormones, the phytoestrogens and related compounds, and the anti-oxidant lycopene, present in tomatoes and some other red plant foods, appear to give protection against some cancers. Other ingredients of vegetarian foods include essential minerals, 'trace

1

elements', and the anti-oxidant vitamins A, C and E. These may add to the protective value of plant food. Another benefit of such diets is that they contain relatively little animal and dairy products, with their high content of animal fat.

For women with breast cancer, early detection and treatment offers the best outcome. Most women with breast cancer will be cured, but the earlier in the disease the cancer is detected and the smaller it is when first treated, the more likely it is that a cure will be achieved.

Regular self-examination and breast-screening programs make a significant difference in detecting breast cancers at an early stage when they are more likely to be curable. Screening programs are based on breast X-rays (mammography), but it is good if they also include breast examination by an expert and facilities for needle biopsy of any suspicious lump or other unusual change in the breast. It is an added advantage if the breast-screening unit has facilities for ultrasound studies.

Once cancer has been detected, the most appropriate course of treatment should be planned by the family doctor and surgeon or a larger medical treatment team, with the patient taking part in the decision making. This is especially important when there is a choice of apparently equally effective approaches to treatment.

Treatment choices may include surgery, radiotherapy, chemo-therapy or management with hormones, or a combination of these. The most appropriate treatment will depend upon the stage of advancement and the degree of abnormality (anaplasia) of the cancer cells. Of most significance is whether or not the cancer has spread into nearby lymph nodes, most often in the armpit, or whether or not the cancer has spread into other organs or tissues distant from the breast area. Other important factors that must be considered are the age and general fitness of the patient, facilities available for immediate and long-term care, and the wishes of the patient. For most patients, it is also important to ascertain, discuss and consider the attitudes of such people as her husband or partner or close family and friends.

The physical needs, as well as the personal concerns, anxieties and attitudes of each individual patient must be acknowledged and taken into consideration. Her regular family doctor should be part of the treatment team, but help will also be needed in physiotherapy, rehabilitation, and, where necessary, in choice of the most appropriate breast prosthesis or breast reconstruction.

Most importantly, support of an understanding counsellor, psychologist, psychiatrist or spiritual adviser can be of inestimable value in helping the patient, her family and friends adjust to the new personal, social, spiritual and economic concerns and anxieties associated with the cancer.

The good news is:

- Most patients with breast cancer are now cured.
- More and more cancers are now being detected at a curable stage.
- In most cases it is not necessary to remove the whole breast to achieve the best treatment results.
- With modern plastic surgery, it is now usually possible to reconstruct a breast of very good appearance for those patients who have had a breast removed.
- It appears that the incidence of breast cancer in women of Western countries during the twentieth century has now passed its peak and is starting to decrease.
- Modern research is leading to constant improvements in both early detection of breast cancer at a curable stage, and better treatment.
- It now appears possible that the risk of developing breast cancer might be reduced by relatively simple means, including by paying attention to diet.

1

Structure and function of the breast

All mammals, that is animals that breast-feed their young, have breasts or mammary glands. In embryonic life in both males and females, cells develop to form a nipple. Fifteen to twenty small rudimentary ducts grow down from the nipple into underlying tissues. The ends of these ducts expand into lobular buds like tiny pouches, and it is these that have the potential to secrete milk.

In males, the breast normally remains as this rudimentary organ under the nipple. Occasionally, in both males and females, a rudimentary third or fourth breast can be present below the nipple line, lower on the chest or abdominal wall. It is rare for such a rudimentary breast to consist of anything more than a small nipple, called an 'accessory nipple', and often this is mistaken for a mole.

In females at puberty, the breast tissue develops further under the influence of female hormones. The ducts grow, enlarge and branch, and the nipple enlarges. Strands of fibrous tissue and globules of fat develop in the breasts, giving them their characteristic shape. Some women develop more of this breast tissue than others, and sometimes a little more tissue is developed in one breast than the other so that one breast is larger than the other. It is perfectly normal for the breasts not to be exactly equal in size.

The ducts and lobular buds undergo changes with each menstrual cycle, preparing for possible pregnancy and breast-feeding, and the breasts swell. If a pregnancy occurs, the ducts and lobules develop further in preparation for milk secretion. If there is no

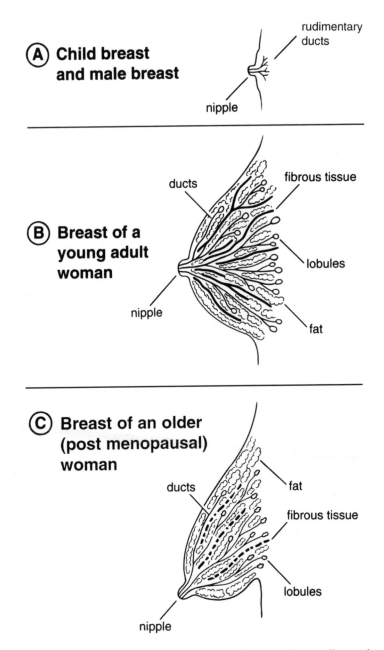

Figure 1.1 (a) Primitive (undeveloped) breast tissue as it normally remains in males and as it is in females before puberty. (b) The breast tissue of a young adult woman, between puberty and menopause. (c) Breast tissue of an older, post-menopausal woman.

pregnancy and menstruation takes place, the changes and swelling reverse and the breasts return to their normal resting state.

After menopause the lobular gland tissue decreases and the fibrous tissue loses its strength, so the breasts lose their firmness. Because they are now composed of proportionally more soft fat, they tend to hang rather lower.

The relative decrease in firm fibrous tissue with relative increase in fat content after menopause means that X-rays are more able to penetrate the breast. This means that mammography of a post-menopausal woman is more likely to be able to show any abnormality and is more likely to be helpful in detecting a firm change in breast tissue that might be a cancer than is mammography of younger women with firmer breasts.

Some women are more aware of the monthly changes in the breast than others, as the breasts can become uncomfortable or even painful. These changes take place in each menstrual cycle over a period of 30 or 40 years, so it is not surprising that sometimes the changes are incomplete and abnormalities such as cysts or lumps can develop in the breasts. Such abnormal developments in the breasts are common during the reproductory years, but they are not cancer and do not lead to cancer. They become more common as the menopause approaches, but they usually settle after the menopause. However, after the menopause the breasts may remain somewhat lumpy or even a little tender.

The most common cause of breast lumps during the years before menopause is called fibrocystic disease. It is sometimes known by other names, including benign mammary dysplasia, atypical hyperplasia, hormonal mastopathy, fibroadenosis cystica, or 'chronic mastitis'.

If a woman is taking hormone replacement therapy (HRT) after the menopause to relieve symptoms of menopause, lumps of this type might continue to develop in the breasts. Sometimes a cancer might also develop in a woman of this age group. Cystic fibrosis lumps are not cancer but they can be confused with cancer, and it may be difficult to determine whether a breast lump is a cyst or lump from the common breast changes of cystic fibrosis or whether it is a lump due to a cancer. A single lump in a breast in the early reproductive years is usually not a cancer, but a single breast lump in an older woman, especially after the menopause, is more likely to be a cancer.

Hormone replacement therapy (HRT) is not routinely given to every woman following menopause because there can be side-effects. The most significant side-effect is a slightly increased risk of breast cancer in some women, and especially in women who have already had a cancer in one breast. A patient and her doctor must therefore discuss whether her symptoms of menopause justify this very small risk. Certainly if the woman has already had one breast cancer, HRT would not be given unless the symptoms of menopause were very disabling. Under these circumstances an alternative therapy might be considered, such as a naturally occurring plant hormone (phytoestrogen). Some recent studies suggest that standard treatment doses of extracts of these plant hormones, particularly an extract from the red clover plant, are effective in some women without causing toxicity or other side-effects.

$$2$$

What is cancer?

The word cancer is Latin for crab. The condition was called cancer in ancient times because an advanced cancer was compared with a crab having claws reaching out into surrounding tissues. However a cancer, or malignant growth, is now known to be a continuous, purposeless, unwanted, uncontrolled and destructive growth of cells.

To understand the problems of breast cancer, it is important first to understand something about cancers in general. Hence throughout this book some description of cancers in general will be given before special reference is made to breast cancer.

Most normal body tissues like the breast are composed of cells that have the ability to divide or reproduce, but they do so only when there is a need. When this need has been satisfied, they stop reproducing. Cells in some tissues, such as the skin or blood, wear out quickly and are constantly being replaced, but they are replaced only to meet the immediate need of the body. Growth or reproduction of these cells then stops. After injury, cells surrounding the injury site reproduce to replace and repair damaged tissues, but the cell reproduction stops once the injury has been repaired and the wound has healed. There is a 'switch-off' mechanism that stops cells dividing after healing is complete. However, in the case of cancer, the new cells are not needed, and cell reproduction continues for no good reason. Excessive numbers of abnormal cells are produced. There is no switching off mechanism. The abnormal and unwanted cells accumulate and spread into surrounding tissues, causing damage and destruction. The excessive abnormal cancer cells also tend to invade blood vessels and lymph vessels, where they may travel to other parts of the body and establish new damaging colonies of unwanted growing cells. These colonies are called *secondary* or *metastatic* cancers.

A cancer is quite different from an infection. An infection is caused by germs or organisms from outside the body that invade body tissues and cause damage. The body defences recognise the invading germs as being composed of unwanted and damaging foreign invading material. The body defences thus establish protective measures to destroy these foreign invading organisms. Invading cancer cells, on the other hand, are cells that have developed abnormally from the body's own cells. They are thus not recognised by the body's defences as foreign, so they continue to grow and invade without being stopped by the body's natural defences.

Changes in cells and in cell appearance

When a cancer develops, the outline, size, and shape of the cancerous cells may change, but the most important changes are in the nucleus of the cells.

The nucleus determines whether the cell is to be a gland cell, a muscle cell, a blood cell, a breast duct cell, a nerve cell, a brain cell, or some other type of cell. It contains the DNA coding for the genes that make up the central functioning part of the cell and give the cell its special characteristics. These genes are inherited from our parents. Sometimes an abnormal gene is inherited, or sometimes when cells divide during tissue growth or repair some change can take place in a gene (a genetic mutation). These changes can involve genes responsible for cell division, and these changes can sometimes lead to the uncontrolled cell division that we know as cancer.

Cells that grow as a result of abnormal genes look abnormal under the microscope. This abnormal appearance is called *anaplasia*. The greater the degree of anaplasia, or the more abnormal the appearance, the more aggressive and dangerous a cancer is likely to be.

Types of cancer

There are three main types of cancer. The most common cancers are those occurring in gland cells or lining cells. Cancers of lining cells include cancers of skin, ducts or the inside lining of hollow organs. A gland is a tissue that makes a substance, like milk in the breast, gastric juice in the stomach, and saliva in the salivary glands. Gland cancers can occur in these or any other glands. Gland and duct cancers are called *carcinomas*. Cancers that occur in other tissues like fat, muscle, bone, arteries or nerves are known as *sarcomas*. Sarcomas are less common than carcinomas, but like all cancers they are malignant and continue to grow and spread and cause damage. Other types of cancer sometimes start in lymphatic tissue or blood-forming tissue. These are more correctly called lymphomas or leukaemias.

In the breast it is the gland cells and cells lining the ducts that have the greatest risk of growing into cancers. However, as breast tissue also has some non-gland cells like fat cells, fibrous cells, nerve cells and blood vessel cells, occasionally a sarcoma will develop in a breast.

How common is cancer?

Cancer occurs in all societies and in all parts of the world. It affects animals as well as people, and they develop similar cancers, including cancer of the breast. In humans, cancer is known to have been present in ancient times, and it is still present today.

The types of cancer most prevalent in a community vary with the age, sex and race of the people, as well as the geographical, economic and environmental situation and diets and lifestyle habits of the people.

In Western societies, cancer is responsible for about 20 per cent of deaths. In Australia in 1991 it passed coronary artery disease as the leading cause of death. Young people in Western societies are more at risk of dying as a result of accidents in the home or on the roads, but in older people of both sexes cancer is the leading cause of death.

Tables 2.1 and 2.2 (p. 12) summarise the most commonly occurring cancers in Western societies (other than skin cancers) and the cancers that most commonly cause death. Skin cancers are

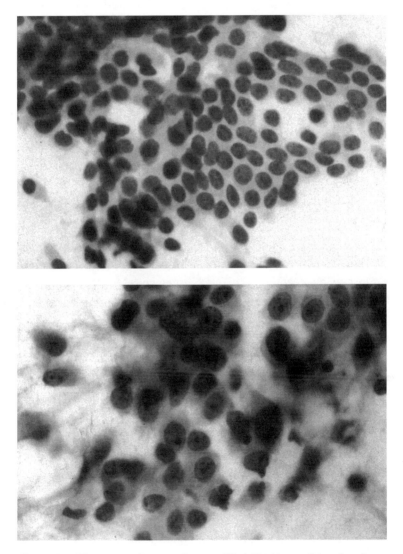

Figure 2.1 Microscope photographs magnified 200 times of (a, above) typical normal breast cells sucked out from an adenoma, a benign (non-malignant) breast lump, and (b, below) anaplastic cancer cells sucked out from a breast cancer. The nucleus shows as a dark centre in the cells. It is much larger and more obvious in the anaplastic cancer cells than in the normal cells.

very common, especially in White people who live in sunny climates but, apart from melanoma, they rarely cause death.

Breast cancer is now the most common cancer (other than skin cancer) of females in most Western societies, although a recent report indicates that lung cancer is now as common in some parts of the US. In Australia, as in most Western societies, the lifetime risk of developing breast cancer is about 1 in 12. That is, it will have occurred in about 1 in 12 women by the age of 75. Until recently it was responsible for more cancer deaths in females than any other cancer because all too often it was not noticed until a well established lump had become obvious. However, lung cancer is less often curable than breast cancer, and lung cancer is now causing more cancer deaths in women in many Western countries.

Table 2.1 Most common cancers in Western countries (other than common skin cancers)

Males	Prostate
Females	Breast
Both sexes together	Large bowel (colon and rectum)
	Lung

Table 2.2 Most common causes of cancer death in Western countries

Males	Lung
Females	Lung
Both sexes together	Lung

Lung cancer is the most common cause of cancer death in men and is probably now the most common cause of cancer death in women. The numbers of women with lung cancer are still increasing, probably because more women have been smoking in recent years. The good news is that the numbers of women with breast cancer and men with prostate and lung cancer appear to have levelled off and have even been decreasing since about 1990.

Breast cancer is about as common in women as active prostate cancer is in men, but the women affected by breast cancer are on average younger than men affected by prostate cancer. In both sexes together in Western societies, bowel cancer is the most common internal cancer and lung cancer is a close second. However, lung cancer is responsible for most cancer deaths in the two sexes together, not only because it is becoming more common, especially in women, but also because in most cases it cannot be cured.

Breast cancer occasionally develops in men in the rudimentary breast ducts under the nipple, but it is rare. Only 1 per cent of breast cancers are in the male breast. When cancer does occur in males it tends to be somewhat more advanced when first diagnosed than it is in females.

Are all tumours in the breast malignant (cancer)?

Benign tumours

Breast lumps are common in adult women of all ages. Most are benign; that is, they are not cancer. In younger women especially, breast lumps are likely to be benign. It is very rare for a benign tumour in the breast to change into a malignant tumour, although it can happen.

Non-malignant or benign tumours are localised collections of cells that seem to be under some sort of control and do not continue to grow or to spread. Although there is no apparent purpose in the growth of benign tumours, the cells in benign tumours are the same, or almost the same, as the cells of the tissue from which they developed. Once a benign tumour reaches a certain size, its growth usually slows down or stops altogether.

Common benign tumours in the breast include benign tumours of gland cells, called adenomas, fibromas in the fibrous tissues of the breast, and a combination type called fibroadenomas. The cells in a breast adenoma look like normal breast cells but they have clumped together as a single lump of cells that is usually covered by a capsule or lining of fibrous tissue. Similarly the cells in a fibroma look like normal fibrous cells that have clumped together. A fibroadenoma is a mixture of both types of cells in a lump, both gland cells and fibrous cells. Adenomas, fibromas or fibroadenomas are not uncommon in the breast. They are usually found as a firm or hard, single, isolated lump, particularly in a breast of younger women in their teens, twenties or thirties. Because these lumps tend to move easily under the fingers when they are being examined, they are sometimes referred to as a 'breast mouse'. As well, softer fatty benign tumours, called lipomas, composed of a lump of normal looking fat cells sometimes occur in the breast. Another benign tumour that is sometimes the cause of a watery or even blood-stained discharge from a nipple is a papilloma in a breast duct. A papilloma is a small fern-like or wart-like benign tumour that grows from the duct wall and projects into the duct.

Any of the tissues of the breast (skin, gland, duct, fat, nerves, muscle, blood vessels or fibrous tissue) can develop either benign or malignant tumours. Almost any lump can develop at almost any age, but the most common are the 'breast mouse' or other benign lumps in younger women, cysts or other lumps of cystic fibrosis in middle-aged women, and malignant lumps of cancer in middle-aged and older women.

The most common cause of breast lumps in women of reproductive age, and especially below the age of 40, is fibrocystic disease. In this condition different types of lumps can develop, such as cysts, fibrous lumps or glandular lumps or a mixture of all three. Sometimes there appears to be just one isolated lump, but more often several lumps can be felt in one or both breasts, or there may be just a general lumpiness felt in one or both breasts. One of the great difficulties with breast lumps is that as women get older towards and past the menopause, breast cancer becomes more common and it is often difficult to decide whether a particular lump is due to cancer or a lump caused by fibrocystic disease.

Malignant tumours

With cancer, or malignant growth, the cells look abnormal and less like the cells from which they developed. Sometimes they are difficult to recognise as breast cells at all. This very abnormal cell appearance, called *anaplasia* (see above), usually gives an indication of the degree of malignancy of the cancer. As a rule, the more malignant the tumour, the more abnormal or *anaplastic* the cells appear. As in any cancer, the division and multiplication of cells continues without control, causing the tumour to get bigger and bigger. It pushes into and grows into surrounding body tissues like skin over the breast or muscle under the breast. Cancer growing through the skin causes ulceration of the skin known as fungation. Cancer growing into underlying muscle becomes firmly attached or fixed to the muscle so that it cannot be moved over the muscle. As cancers grow and invade, there is an increasing risk that they will grow into lymph vessels and blood vessels and other passages and spread to other parts of the body where they establish secondary (metastatic) growths.

Is breast cancer always dangerous?

Cancers are dangerous when they cause damage and destruction to surrounding tissues and when they spread somewhere else and establish secondary (or metastatic) cancers. It is rather like the wind spreading seeds of a weed through a garden. Some will grow in places where they do harm to other plants. The secondary growths of cancer, like the garden weeds, cause damage and destruction to tissues near or around them. Gradually tissues in organs in several different parts of the body might become damaged or destroyed. For example, secondaries in the liver interfere with the function of the liver, and secondaries in the lung block air passages and interfere with breathing, leading to lung infection or pneumonia. Secondaries in the brain will cause pressure on the brain and interfere with brain function, possibly causing headaches, fits or coma. Bones are common sites for secondaries of breast cancer. In bones, secondaries cause pain and weakness of the bones and in some cases the bones may collapse or break.

If any cancer is detected early, while it is still small and before it has spread (metastasised) to another place, it can usually be completely removed surgically, or destroyed in some other way, so that it can be cured before any serious damage has been done. If these early cancers are completely removed before they have spread, the patient will be cured. This is as true of breast cancer as other types of cancer, although the risk that breast cancer will spread is greater than for some other cancers. Even though a breast cancer may seem to be small and confined to the breast, there is still a risk that it may have already spread to other places. The more anaplastic or abnormal-looking the cells, the greater is this risk.

Although small, apparently localised, breast cancers are much less likely to have spread to other places than are bigger, apparently localised, cancers, there is no way of knowing for sure just which cancers will have already spread. Those that do grow and spread into other tissues will sooner or later cause a great deal of distress and eventually death unless they can be controlled.

The best clue as to whether a breast cancer may have spread more widely is whether it has already spread into lymph nodes in the armpit. If a microscopic examination finds no cancer cells in the lymph nodes in the armpit, there is a better than 80 per cent chance that this cancer has not spread beyond its original site in the breast. For a patient with such a cancer, adequate treatment of the breast should give an excellent chance of cure. On the other hand, the more lymph nodes in the armpit that are found to have cancer cells in them, the greater the risk that this cancer will have already spread beyond the armpit and into lung, liver, bone or somewhere else.

The other indication that might suggest that the cancer is more likely to have already spread to other tissues is the degree of abnormal appearance (anaplasia) of the cancer cells as seen under the microscope. Cancer cells that look more like normal breast cells are less likely to spread or metastasise than anaplastic cancer cells that have lost the special features of breast cells and no longer look like breast cells.

Secondary (metastatic) breast cancer

A secondary or metastatic cancer is a cancer that is growing in an organ or tissue some distance away from the tissue or organ in which it originally started. The most important differences between benign tumours and malignant tumours are that benign tumours tend to grow very slowly or not at all, and they stay where they started; that is, they remain localised to the tissue in which they began. Malignant tumours (cancers), on the other hand, tend to continue to grow into and damage surrounding structures. They may also spread into tissues or organs away from the original or primary site where they started. To spread to distant sites, the malignant cells usually grow into blood vessels or lymph vessels, where single cells or small clumps of cells break off and are carried by the bloodstream or the lymphatic vessels to a distant organ or tissue or to lymph nodes. When they have reached a suitable site in a lymph node or other tissue, they may grow as secondary or metastatic tumours. The spreading cancer cells act rather like 'seeds' being transported along blood or lymph vessels to a new 'soil' where they may take root and grow. For some cancers malignant cells may also sometimes spread along nerve sheaths or across body cavities such as the abdominal cavity.

The most common site for metastatic spread of breast cancers is via lymph vessels into lymph nodes. First they most commonly grow in lymph nodes near the breast, especially in the armpit, then spread into lymph nodes in the lower neck or in the chest or further away. With breast cancer the next most common sites of spread are by the bloodstream into bones, lungs or liver. In fact this cancer can spread into almost any organ or tissue, including the other breast, the ovaries, brain, adrenal glands, skin, fat under the skin or to lymph nodes in the abdomen, or almost any part of the body. However, there are some organs and tissues in which metastatic growths rarely develop, for no obvious reason. Like the seeds of a weed growing in a garden, they like to grow in some soils but not so much in others. Breast cancer 'seeds' seem to like to grow especially in lymph nodes, lung, liver and bones, but they rarely take root in muscles or the spleen for some reason not fully understood.

What causes cancer?

For generations doctors, researchers, philosophers, and 'quacks' have been trying to find a single cause for all cancers, and consequently a single cure. No such single cause has been found and probably none exists. However, the different factors causing cancer may all act through a similar or common pathway, in that one way or another they affect the genes in cells, and the genes are responsible for the division and growth of cells. So it is that a range of cancer-causing factors that can be grouped in categories such as environment, smoking, diet, age, race, hormones, and social customs can all eventually affect genes. The genes (inherited from our parents) are in the nucleus of cells, and these genes are responsible for growing new cells for growth or repair or replacement of worn-out cells. It is the genes that cause dividing cells to grow as needed for special purposes in different parts of the body.

In this chapter the known categories of cancer-causing factors will be outlined. We conclude with an account of how changes in genes might result in a cancer developing.

Environmental associations

Many common cancers can be traced to known causes or be associated with environmental conditions. For example, exposure to ultraviolet light in sunshine is directly or indirectly responsible for most skin cancers. Tobacco causes cancers in many tissues—lungs, mouth, throat and larynx, as well as the oesophagus, stomach, pancreas, kidney, bladder and even the breast. The human papilloma virus can cause cancer of the cervix, vagina or vulva in women, the penis in men, and the skin in either sex. Other viruses, such as Hepatitis B, Hepatitis C, and the AIDS virus, can be indirect causes of other cancers. Some cancers can be related to 'recreational' drugs—marijuana as well as tobacco with lung cancer, and betel nut with mouth cancer. Certain industrial carcinogens (such as excessive soot, asbestos, benzene, aniline dyes, phosphorus, arsenic, some wood and metal chippings) and some air pollutants have been incriminated in other cancers. Some forms of irradiation, such as the high doses of X-rays that were commonly given when X-rays were first used, and exposure to radiation from atomic bombs, have also been incriminated as causes of cancer.

Neither short-term follow-up studies of survivors of atomic bomb irradiation nor short-term studies of women smokers have shown any increase in breast cancer. However, long-term studies show there is an increased risk of breast cancer after many years of smoking, particularly in women who began smoking in the developing years of puberty or younger. Recent evidence also indicates that passive smoking may be a significant risk factor—there appears to be an increased risk in women who were brought up in households where one or both parents were smokers. Increased numbers of people with breast cancer have also been seen in long-term follow-up studies of women who were exposed as girls to irradiation in the atomic bombings of Hiroshima and Nagasaki. However, neither smoking nor irradiation are responsible for the majority of breast cancers.

Smoking

The habit of smoking outweighs all other known influences as a cause of serious cancer in present-day men and women. The incidence of lung cancer is some eight to ten times higher in smokers than non-smokers, and the risk is directly related to the amount of tobacco smoked and inhaled.

The relationship of tobacco smoking to breast cancer is not as close as it is for a lot of other cancers. However, women who have smoked for 30 years or more do have an increased risk. This is most apparent in women who began smoking when very young, especially if they started at or before the age of puberty.

Diet

A good balanced diet means different things in different countries and in different cultural traditions. However, in any society good balanced diets should include adequate protein for body building, carbohydrate and some fat (preferably not animal fat) mainly for energy, a full range of vitamins, and a good balance of minerals. Healthy bowel and good bowel activity also require abundant fibre. Good dietary habits should be encouraged from childhood to give the best chances of prolonged good health. Obesity should be avoided. Daily exercise should be part of a continuous lifestyle program for good health, and harmful products like tobacco or excessive alcohol should be avoided.

There is an association between diet and some cancers of the digestive tract. Certainly a high-fibre diet appears to be protective against bowel cancer. The differences between Asians and Westerners in the incidences of other cancers, especially differences in the incidence of breast and prostate cancers, may also be related to diet. Traditionally Asians have a diet with a high content of legumes (peas, lentils, soya beans etc.). Of all plant foods, legumes have the greatest amounts of naturally occurring plant hormones, the *phytoestrogens*, and in particular their most active components called *isoflavones*. Studies suggest that these dietary ingredients may be most significant in the relatively low incidence of breast cancer in Asian females and relatively low incidence of prostate cancer in Asian males. Asian women also have a lower incidence of other breast problems as well as cancer.

With the increased affluence of the industrial revolution about 200 years ago, many Europeans changed from simple peasant diets, high in legumes and other plant foods, to diets much higher in animal products. It appears that the incidence of breast diseases, including cancer, among Europeans was less before Western diets changed in this way.

There are so many variable factors in different population groups that it is always difficult to prove which particular factors may have caused any difference in the incidence of cancer. For most cancers, other than breast and prostate cancers and cancers of the digestive passages and digestive organs, diet is probably not significant.

Fats in the diet

A high intake of animal fat may be associated with increased risk of breast cancer, particularly if the habit was started in childhood. However, there is also evidence that the fat of olive oil might have some protective value. It seems that saturated fats (mainly animal fats) and even polyunsaturated fats (present in most margarines) may slightly increase breast cancer risk, but monounsaturated fats (plentiful in olive oil) are possibly protective. Women of southern European and Mediterranean countries where olive oil is a regular ingredient of diets have a rather lower incidence of breast cancer than women in northern European countries who are more likely to have diets higher in animal fats. Part of the explanation may be that olive oil gives some protection against breast cancer.

Vegetarian diets

A diet high in plant foods and low in animal fats does appear to offer protection. Members of the Seventh Day Adventist Church, who are vegetarians, have a lower than average incidence of breast cancers; they also have a lower incidence of a number of other cancers including cancers of the oesophagus, stomach, pancreas, colon and rectum, prostate and lung. However, as well as being vegetarians with a high fibre diet and low consumption of meat and animal fat, these people are usually strictly monogamous, non-smokers, and do not drink alcohol. These and other differences in lifestyles may well be more significant, especially with such cancers as lung cancer. A reduced incidence of breast cancer has been reported in those church members who practise strict vegetarianism with no intake of animal products, not even eggs or dairy products.

Obesity

Women who are distinctly overweight have a greater risk of breast cancer than thin women. Whether this is directly associated with obesity or more closely associated with diet is uncertain. Certainly overweight people are usually those who eat diets with more animal fat and diets with less dependence on fresh fruits, vegetables, legumes, nuts, unprocessed grains and other plant foods. They are also less likely to keep fit with regular active exercise. These dietary and other factors are possibly of more relevance to breast cancer than the actual body weight of the women.

Alcohol

Moderate alcohol consumption (no more than one or two drinks a day) is not associated with increased risk of breast cancer. However, heavy alcohol consumption has been associated with an increased risk of breast cancer, as well as with an increased incidence of cancer of the mouth and throat, oesophagus, stomach, liver, and pancreas.

Who is at special risk?

Pre-existing tumours

In a lot of other cancers the cancer might have developed from a pre-existing benign (harmless) tumour or other pre-existing benign or harmless abnormality. It was once believed that this might also have been true of breast cancer but it has not been found to be the case. Pre-existing fibrocystic disease has not been found to be significant as a precursor of breast cancer. However, both fibrocystic disease and breast cancer are common in middle-aged women of Western societies, so both conditions may be present in the same patient.

History of a previous cancer

People who have been cured of one cancer often ask about the risk of developing a second cancer. While it is true that some people have an increased predisposition towards developing cancer, in most cases the increased risk of getting a second serious cancer is not great.

There is no evidence that women who have previously been treated for another type of cancer have any greater or lesser risk of subsequently getting breast cancer, with the exception of a small increased risk for women who have previously had ovarian cancer. Women who have been treated for cancer in one breast do have an increased risk of developing cancer in the other breast, although by far the majority of women do not develop a second cancer. They also have an increased risk of developing a further cancer in the affected breast if the breast was not totally removed, but again most women do not develop a further cancer. This increased risk is real but not great. Most women do not get a further cancer.

Is there an inherited risk?

In some relatively uncommon cancers there is a strong hereditary factor, and in other cancers there is a less obvious hereditary factor. For most cancers there is no evidence of a hereditary factor at all. Among the cancers with a strong hereditary factor is a condition called 'familial polyposis coli', in which half the children of an affected parent are likely to develop multiple polyps in the large bowel. A particular oncogene—a gene that can cause cancer—inherited from an affected parent is responsible for this abnormality, which causes affected people to develop cancer in the bowel, usually by about the age of 40.

Breast cancer is one of the more common cancers with an increased familial incidence. Women are at slightly greater risk if they have a close relative such as a mother or sister who has had a breast cancer. The risk is further increased in women with two close relatives who have had the disease. What is responsible for this apparent increased risk in some families is not always clear. It may be strictly an inherited oncogene that affects the cells, tissues or body defences, or it may be that members of these families are more likely to have similar dietary habits or be affected by other similar environmental conditions.

The increased risk for relatives of sufferers is small in most families, but in occasional families there may be a considerably increased risk. For example, there have been rare reports of families in which about half the female blood relatives have developed breast cancer. In such families it is likely that an aberrant gene or oncogene is at least partly responsible. Two aberrant genes called BRCA 1 and BRCA 2 have now been discovered and are found to be responsible for some families having increased risk of breast cancer. (The name BRCA is contrived from BReast CAncer.) Breast cancer in women under the age of 40 is more likely to be associated with an aberrant gene than is breast cancer in older women. For the majority of women with breast cancer, other factors appear to be more significant, especially absence of pregnancies or possibly interrupted pregnancies, and other hormonal factors associated with years of fertility and menstruation. There also appears to be an association with diet.

Although breast cancer in men is uncommon, when it does occur there might be a familial association. Some breast cancers in men are linked to inheritance of the BRCA 2 gene.

Age

In general, the risk of developing most cancers increases with age. Breast cancer is uncommon in women before the age of 40 and very uncommon before the age of 30, although no age is exempt and a few cases have even been seen in teenagers. After the age of 40 the incidence increases, with a peak age group at about 60 years. Statistically about 1 per cent occur before the age of 30 and about 10 per cent occur before the age of 50. However, by far the majority (90 per cent) of breast cancers are first seen in women over the age of 50.

Breast cancer is very uncommon in girls and young women under the age of 30, but carcinogenic influences appear to have a greater effect on breast tissue during the early years of breast development. For example, early studies showed that women exposed to atomic irradiation at Hiroshima and Nagasaki subsequently developed increased numbers of several cancers such as leukaemias, lymphomas and thyroid cancer, but in the short-term studies only a few years after the bombing they were not found to have an obvious increased risk of breast cancer. Some years later, however, it was found that women who suffered this irradiation exposure as young girls did have an increased risk of breast cancer in their later years. Recent studies have also shown that girls brought up in a home where parents have been smokers have an increased risk of developing breast cancer later in life. It appears that the influence of passive smoking, like the influence of atomic irradiation, is significant in girls when their breasts are developing during infancy and childhood but especially during puberty. Studies have also shown that there is an increased breast cancer risk in women who began a smoking habit when they were very young.

Hormonal activity, HRT and the Pill

There is a clear relationship between a woman's hormonal activity and risk of developing breast cancer. Women who begin to menstruate early in life (around 10 or 12 years of age) and have menopause late in life (possibly at the age of 50 or more) have a greater risk of developing breast cancer than women who have fewer years of potentially fertile hormonal activity. Having babies early in life and possibly prolonged breast-feeding and having several babies appear to be protective. This protection may be because these events reduce the number of unproductive hormonal menstrual cycles.

Women who take female hormones (oestrogens) as hormone replacement therapy (HRT) to reduce post-menopausal symptoms (PMS) are known to have a slightly increased risk of developing breast cancer. The contraceptive pills first used in the 1960s are also found to be associated with a small increased risk of breast cancer. However, the low dose oestrogen–progesterone contraceptive pills now used appear to have no increased risk and may even have some protective value. There have been inconclusive suggestions from some studies that women who have had interrupted pregnancies (that is, abortions) may have a slightly increased risk of developing breast cancer later.

Other causes

Does race play a part?

Some cancers are more prevalent in people of some races than in other races. Whether the most significant factor is genetic or racial or whether it is more likely due to environment, habits, diet or other influences is hard to determine. Some examples of increased racial incidence are a higher incidence of stomach cancer in Japan and Korea, a higher incidence of cancer of the oesophagus in certain African ethnic groups, and a high incidence of liver cancer (hepatoma) in Malaysians and Africans. In Israel, a country with one of the highest incidences of thyroid cancer, the disease is more common amongst Jews born in Europe than in those born in Asia. In South Africa, Bantus have a much higher incidence of thyroid cancer than do Blacks from other regions.

Breast cancer is certainly more common in women of 'developed countries', like the UK, western Europe, the US, Canada, Australia and New Zealand. The high incidence of breast cancer in women, prostate cancer in men and large bowel cancer in both sexes in Europeans and people of European descent has caused these three cancers to be called 'the Western cancers'. However, the high incidence is not confined to the Caucasian (White) women in these countries. Social customs (including motherhood), diet and other factors appear to be more significant than race.

In regard to breast cancer, the incidence increased in Western societies during the twentieth century. It has remained much lower in those Asians and Africans who have continued to live in their traditional lifestyles in Asia and Africa. Women of Asian or African ethnic background who have adopted Western lifestyles in Western countries have an increased incidence of breast cancer similar to their fellow citizens of Caucasian ethnic backgrounds. It seems therefore that race is not of great significance in breast cancer and may not be significant at all. While there are genetic influences that predispose people of different races to develop different cancers, it is hard to know with any particular cancer whether the most significant factors are genetic or due to something else the people have in common. Social habits or diet or sometimes economic or other influences, or a combination of a number of different factors, may be of greater significance.

Cultural and social customs

There is a relationship between the development of some cancers, including breast cancer, and cultural and social customs. Apart from diet, the most obvious of these relationships is the age at which women have their first babies and possibly the number of babies they have, whether they breast-feed their babies and, if so, for how long. The most consistent of these relationships is that women who have their first baby when quite young and possibly as teenagers have a distinctly lower risk of getting a breast cancer than do women who have never had a baby or who have their first baby late in life. Having several babies and prolonged breast-feeding may also reduce breast cancer risk.

The wearing of bras

There have been reports that the wearing of bras might increase the risk of breast cancer, but there is no conclusive evidence to support this theory. Bras are less commonly worn by women in 'undeveloped' countries, where other factors mean that women have a relatively lower risk of breast cancer. Strong tight bras are more likely to be worn by overweight women, and overweight women have a slightly increased risk, but there is no evidence that the wearing of a bra is responsible for any increased cancer risk. As a general health measure, women are better advised not to wear excessively tight bras that may irritate or cause pressure damage.

Breast implants

Breast implants have received a good deal of publicity and criticism in the press, but there is no evidence to incriminate implants as a cause of breast cancer. However, it is true that it may be more difficult to detect a cancer in a breast containing an implant, so there could be some delay in diagnosing and treating cancer in a breast that has an implant in it.

Does geography or environment play a part?

The incidence of a particular type of cancer varies from country to country and even varies within the one country according to geographic and other conditions. However, as previously noted, it is often difficult to be sure whether the difference is essentially due to different geographical and climatic elements or to race, to lifestyle differences, or possibly to combinations of these.

The association of skin cancer and melanoma with fair-skinned people living in a sunny climate is obvious. The incidence is highest in fair-skinned people living in sunny climates in Australia and in the sunny southern parts of the United States.

The association between the high incidence of breast cancer in Europe, North America, Australia and New Zealand and the much lower incidence in India, China, Japan and other Asian and African countries appears not to be especially related to race or geography. There is a closer association with lifestyle practices and especially the diets of the citizens of these countries. When they move to Western countries or adopt Western diets and lifestyle practices, the risk of breast cancer in women of Asian or African ethnic origin becomes similar to that of other Western women.

Is occupation significant?

There is no convincing evidence of any significant association between occupation and breast cancer apart from links with the other practices associated with the occupation. For example, practising nuns have a higher than average incidence of breast cancer, but this is much more likely to be associated with the fact that they do not have babies or breast-feed babies rather than the occupation itself.

Previous sexual behaviour

There is no evidence of a relationship between previous sexual behaviour and breast cancer, other than a lower risk in women who have had babies early in life and breast-fed them. They have a lower risk than women who have never had a baby or who had a first baby when nearing or past the age of 40.

AIDS, hepatitis and other viruses

There is no evidence that in the normal course of events any cancer can be passed from one individual to another. AIDS (acquired immune deficiency syndrome) is caused by a virus infection that may predispose sufferers to cancer because it damages natural immune defences. AIDS patients have lowered resistance to infections and are more prone to some forms of cancer, but there is no particular association with breast cancer. Liver cancer is not infectious, but a common cause of liver cancer is infection with the hepatitis B or hepatitis C viruses. These hepatitis infections spread easily from person to person, mainly from food or intimate contact, and liver cancer develops more commonly in people who have been infected. The human papilloma virus is often a sexually transmitted infection, and can cause cancer of the cervix, vagina or vulva in women or cancer of the penis in men, as well as skin cancers, but no association has been seen with breast cancer. There is no evidence of any relationship between breast cancer and any infection.

Psychological or emotional factors

Amongst the more unusual theories for causes of cancer is the suggestion that, like emotional and some mental (psychosomatic) illnesses, cancer may result from an unnatural suppression of the 'fight or flight' response to anxiety or stress. It has been suggested that if a stressful situation persists over a long period and the person concerned feels that whatever action he or she takes will be wrong, a subconscious decision to escape through death by cancer may result. There is little evidence to support such a theory, although some retrospective studies have indicated that a high proportion of cancer patients have experienced some form of severe stress in the period six months to two years before the onset of illness.

Most psychologists would not claim that psychological reactions are a direct cause of cancer, but some feel that they may play a part alongside known chemical, genetic, environmental, dietary, degenerative, viral or radiation causes. Certainly, the association of possible psychological factors with cancer and the worry and emotional reaction of hearing a diagnosis of cancer has indicated a need for additional psychological support for many patients. Such support may be best given by psychiatrists, clinical psychologists, social workers or other trained health workers. For some patients an understanding member of the clergy or other spiritual adviser can be most helpful.

For any patient with a cancer the need for psychological adjustment has long been recognised by a variety of alternative medicine practitioners. This need, often unfulfilled, is given as a reason for their practices of treatment by faith healing, meditation and even, in some cases, for a variety of herbal or other unproven nontraditional or pseudo-medical therapies. Because of the special social and sexual association of the breast, virtually all women diagnosed with breast cancer have special psychological and spiritual needs for understanding, and this need may continue for years after the initial treatment. However, there is no evidence to suggest that such deep emotions were responsible for causing the cancer, as has been proposed by some alternative health practitioners.

The best clues

In summary, the most apparent common association with breast cancer is cellular degeneration associated with increasing age and with hormonal activity causing repeated and uninterrupted cell changes over many years. This is most apparent in women who have had no pregnancies to interrupt their hormonal breast changes every month over many years. Other associations may be familial or genetic, possibly racial, and possibly geographic. Some carcinogenic influences like active smoking, passive smoking or ionising irradiation apparently have a much greater potential to damage developing breast tissue early in life or during puberty than later in life, although the breast cancer is more likely to develop some years later. There is strong suspicion that diet is significant, and it also appears that the earlier in life good dietary habits are started the greater their benefit.

Genetic factors and gene changes

It is not known whether the different cancer-causing factors described above all activate biological 'triggers' in cells. Possibly changes in genes in the cells stimulate the cells to reproduce indiscriminately and so become a cancer. Another possibility is that the cancer factors just weaken the body defences against cells that continue to divide. A third possibility is that they interfere with the body's natural ability to apply a braking mechanism to cell growth. This braking mechanism appears to be an inbuilt quality of cells that not only acts to stop them dividing but which also makes them 'self-destruct' after they have served their useful period of life. This inbuilt self-destruction when they are no longer needed is called *apoptosis*. Recent studies suggest a combination of these theories might be correct—an accelerated growth of new cells, loss or failure of the braking mechanism that stops new cells from dividing, and loss of protection against abnormal new cells. Whatever the mechanism or combination of mechanisms, it seems that cancers are ultimately caused by changes in genes or *proto-oncogenes* that convert them into *oncogenes*, genes that can cause cancer.

Oncogenes

The many functions of our body cells are controlled by genes, coded in the DNA that makes up the chromosomes or genetic library of our cells. Like the genes that determine things like eye colour and hair colour and blood group, we inherit these controlling genes from our parents, and there is some evidence of a link between genetic make-up and some cancers.

All cells contain special genes called *proto-oncogenes*. These proto-oncogenes are responsible for switching on the self-limiting repair process when a tissue is injured or its cells are worn out and need to be replaced. When the repair is complete, the healing mechanism is switched off. The cancer-causing agents may cause the proto-oncogenes to change into potentially cancer-causing *oncogenes*. Oncogenes can result from a number of factors as previously discussed, including action of some viruses, action of chemical carcinogens, irradiation, and sometimes what appears to be *spontaneous genetic mutation*. Genetic mutation is a change in cells arising from the action of one of the cancer-causing agents, or it can be spontaneous, arising from an apparent accidental change during cell division. Particularly in older people, after so many billion cell divisions to keep the body in good function and repair, it is little wonder that an accident can occasionally happen in the division of cells. The real wonder is that it does not happen more often, even if we do avoid carcinogens and keep our bodies in good shape. It is certainly little wonder that genetic accidents happen if we expose our cells to known carcinogens like tobacco or radiation, or don't provide our tissues with good nourishment by providing what they need in our diets, but sometimes genetic mutation accidents just happen without any apparent cause.

When an oncogene is active in a cell, the nature of the life-giving DNA of the cell is changed so that the switched-on mechanism of growth and repair continues instead of being switched off as it should be, and the cells that are produced do not undergo apoptosis (self-destruction) when they are no longer needed.

Some people inherit abnormal oncogenes from their parents, but in the majority of people who develop cancer something happening later in life has changed normal inherited proto-oncogenes into oncogenes. These changed proto-oncogenes or sometimes inherited oncogenes predispose those affected to a greater risk of cancer. So the cancer-causing oncogenes may be inherited at conception, or result from cancer-causing agents changing proto-oncogenes into oncogenes, or result from accidental genetic mutation of dividing cells at times of cell growth or after the many years of cell division during the course of a normal life, a risk that increases with age.

Recent studies have shown that hereditary breast cancer may result from changes (mutation) in one of several specific genes that have been inherited from a parent, but it is thought that less than 10 per cent of breast cancers result from an abnormal inherited gene.

Male breast cancer

Because it is very uncommon, it is difficult to find information about associations or causes of breast cancer in men. The average age for men with breast cancer is about eight or ten years older than for women. Breast cancer in men has become a little more common in recent years, but the increase is not nearly as obvious as in women. Studies have not found any particular dietary or racial associations. The only significant finding so far detected is a genetic association with the BRCA 2 gene in some cases.

4

Can breast cancer be prevented?

There is no definite answer to the question 'Can breast cancer be prevented?' The most accepted protection against death from breast cancer is its detection and removal in its earliest stages, especially pre-invasive 'in situ' breast cancer before it has become 'invasive' (see chapter 5). However, the most promising and practical approaches to potential prevention of breast cancer in the first place are hormone modification, possibly with an anti-hormone like tamoxifen, dietary approaches, and avoiding smoking.

Anti-hormones—tamoxifen

There is no known way of making any individual immune to the development of cancer. Theoretically the only sure way to prevent breast cancer totally would be to remove both breasts early in life, but obviously to the vast majority of women and communities this would be unthinkable. The next most certain way, but also unthinkable, would be to get rid of the hormones known to be associated with stimulation of breast changes and breast cancer; that is, the female hormones produced by the ovaries. To remove both ovaries early in life is again unacceptable, but it does leave an idea that can be acted upon by women at particular risk later in life.

Studies have shown that if the anti-oestrogen agent *tamoxifen* is given to women at high risk of breast cancer to reduce the effect of their natural hormones, this does reduce their risk of later developing a breast cancer. This protection is now being used for women at special risk such as women with a strong family history of breast cancer or women who have previously had a breast cancer, but only after they have had all the children they wish to have. The gain in having a lower risk of breast cancer is to some extent counterbalanced by a slightly greater risk of a less common cancer, cancer of the body of the uterus, later in life. However, a woman at very high risk of developing breast cancer may well be justified in taking a small daily dose of tamoxifen or a similar product that stops the action of her own hormones in stimulating breast tissue.

Diet and breast cancer

Many researchers now believe there is important potential for reducing the risk of developing breast cancer by learning some lessons from the dietary practices of those races, communities or countries with a low incidence of this cancer. Studies are presently being conducted to determine whether diet can change the incidence of breast cancer.

There is a lot of evidence to indicate that women who adhere to a vegetarian diet will have a reduced risk of breast cancer. There are two main theoretical reasons for this. First is the high content of plant hormones in vegetarian diets, especially the isoflavone types of phytoestrogens and related compounds. These are particularly plentiful in peas, beans and other legumes, but especially in soya beans. It seems that plant oestrogens compete with and block the action of the woman's own oestrogens, resulting in a much weaker stimulation of breast tissue than uninterrupted stimulation by the woman's own oestrogens.

There are a number of rather different phytoestrogens in plant foods, but there are two main groups. These are the *lignans*, present in small amounts in all plants and especially nuts, grains and berries, and the *isoflavones*, present in all legumes. Peas, beans and especially soya beans contain relatively large quantities of isoflavones. Of this group of phytoestrogens, all the most active isoflavones are present in greatest concentration in the red clover plant. The red clover does not feature in either Eastern or Western human diets, but tablets are now available that contain in one tablet as much of the isoflavones as is consumed in a traditional Asian daily diet. Australian-produced red clover tablets have been designed specifically for this purpose. Studies are presently being conducted to determine whether by taking a daily dose of these tablets (one to three tablets daily depending on the brand) the risk of breast cancer and other breast problems can be reduced in women who otherwise have a traditional Western diet.

Laboratory studies have confirmed that breast cancer cells become fewer in number and less aggressive and apparently less dangerous after exposure to preparations made from isoflavones. A second proposal is for Western women to adopt a completely vegetarian diet with a high soy content, including the use of soy milk. However, this suggestion is unlikely to be adhered to by most Westerners, and such a diet is possibly no more beneficial than a diet with reduced animal fat combined with one, two or three small tablets daily.

Vitamins, anti-oxidants and trace elements

Dietary advice often gives special emphasis to 'protective' vitamins and especially the anti-oxidant vitamins A, C and E.

Anti-oxidants are believed to inactivate toxic substances that accumulate in the body after normal body activity, and are often mentioned in relation to breast cancer. So too is the element selenium, present in small quantities in most plants and especially in nuts and grains, and in fish, eggs and meat—provided the soils where these are produced are not themselves deficient in selenium.

As yet there is no convincing evidence that taking additional vitamins or selenium over and above basic requirements does anything special, but there is also no evidence that they do not. At this stage the best advice is that a *little* extra can do no harm and might be of some benefit, so why not. However, there can be too much of a good thing, as very large doses of vitamin A can be damaging and excess selenium can be toxic.

Lycopenes

Recent dietary studies, especially from Harvard Medical School in the US and from Israel, have shown evidence of a possible protective link between certain cancers and the anti-oxidant *lycopene*, the red colouring ingredient of tomatoes and some other red fruits and vegetables. Lycopene can now be produced in commercial quantities from tomatoes. Laboratory studies, as well as both human and animal studies, suggest that it may protect against a number of degenerative diseases including heart disease, eye degeneration and some cancers, including breast cancer. Tissue culture and other studies suggest that lycopene may help prevent some cancers or inhibit the growth of some cancer cells, including breast and prostate cancer cells. When lycopene is combined with certain B and D vitamins these anti-cancer effects appear to be increased. Further studies are now being made to discover whether isoflavones and lycopene together have a greater (synergistic) effect than the sum of the effects of these two compounds given separately.

Lycopene appears to be better absorbed from cooked tomatoes or tomato pastes or tomato sauces than from fresh raw tomatoes or tomato juice. This can be good news to those who like to smother foods with tomato sauces or pastes. However, until more studies are complete the only conclusion is to reinforce the value of certain natural foods in the diet, including tomatoes and tomato products.

Smoking

The most obvious preventive measure in reducing the risk of developing many serious cancers is to avoid smoking. The relationship between smoking and breast cancer has not been as apparent as with many other cancers, but after many years of smoking there is an increased risk of breast cancer, especially if the smoking habit began at or before puberty. Obviously for this reason alone it is best not to smoke, although the health risks of smoking extend to many more diseases and health problems than breast cancer alone.

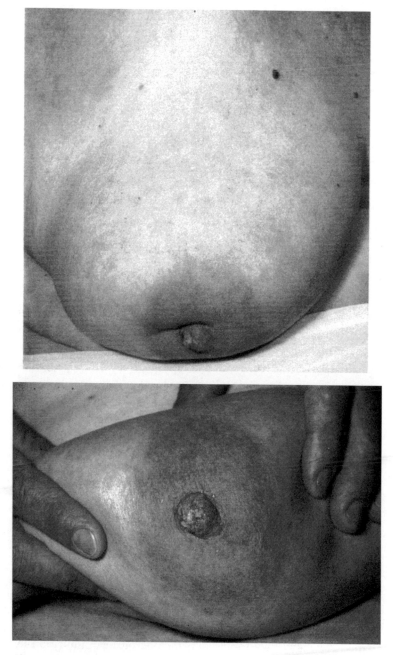

Figure 5.3 (a, above) A recently inverted nipple and (b, below) Paget's disease of the nipple. In both cases cancer was found under the nipple area.

Occasionally the first evidence of a breast cancer, like other cancers, can be general symptoms like malaise (tiredness and feeling unwell), lethargy and loss of energy, loss of appetite, weight loss or the effects of anaemia. However the effect of spread of secondaries to other organs such as lungs or liver is rarely the first indication of breast cancer.

Two important measures are advocated for women in the breast cancer age groups to improve their chances of detecting a possible breast cancer at the earliest and most curable stage. These are regular self-examination, and professional screening tests.

Self-examination of the breasts

All adult women should get into the habit of self-examination of their breasts. A good routine is to make a point of examining the breasts with wet soapy fingers in the bath or shower once each month, preferably after the completion of menstruation when the breasts should have settled down from possible pre-menstrual engorgement. There are several simple routine techniques for self-examination of the breasts and armpit regions. Small pamphlets available from most doctors' surgeries, hospitals, breast clinics, cancer societies or other special cancer organisations can help each woman find a routine that is most appropriate and comfortable for her.

Screening tests

Regular screening tests are recommended for women in the most likely breast cancer age group, that is women over the age of about 45 to 50, and for younger women in a high risk group, such as women with a strong family history of breast cancers. These screening tests are usually arranged in special breast cancer screening clinics, sometimes in mobile clinics, or sometimes in major hospitals. They are based on special breast X-rays called mammograms. Preferably they should also include breast examination by an experienced clinician and it is good to have ultrasound facilities, although these are not regarded as essential components of initial breast screening clinics.

It is most important for screening clinics to have access to biopsy facilities if any lump or other suspicious area is found. In the most common biopsy technique, a needle and syringe is used to suck out (aspirate) some cells from the lump or abnormal area. The cells sucked out in this way are examined microscopically to look for abnormal cells that may be evidence of cancer.

A lump in the male breast

In men a lump under a nipple is usually more obvious than a breast lump in a woman, especially in a woman who has big breasts. However, men are usually more reluctant to seek medical advice for a breast lump. Fortunately most such lumps in a male breast are benign. They are usually due to duct and glandular enlargement sometimes associated with hormonal changes in men. Occasionally, however, a lump in a man's breast is a cancer that behaves in a similar way to a cancer in a woman's breast.

Mammograms

There is no single absolutely reliable screening test to diagnose the presence of breast cancer. *Mammograms* are the most helpful and the most commonly used screening test for possible breast cancer. They are non-invasive, meaning the test can be performed without cutting into or otherwise taking a piece of tissue from the breast.

Mammograms are simply specialised X-ray studies in which very small doses of X-rays are used to show the underlying breast tissue on X-ray film or on a TV screen. X-rays penetrate some tissues more easily than others, and pass through air easily. X-rays make the underlying film darker when they pass through air than when they try to penetrate more solid structures like fibrous tissue or cartilage. Bones and metals cannot be penetrated by X-rays, so they leave no effect on the underlying X-ray films. These materials thus make shadows that appear as white areas on the film. Fat and muscle are fairly easily penetrated, but fibrous tissue or cancer tissue is less easily penetrated and may show as lighter areas on a film than fat or muscle do.

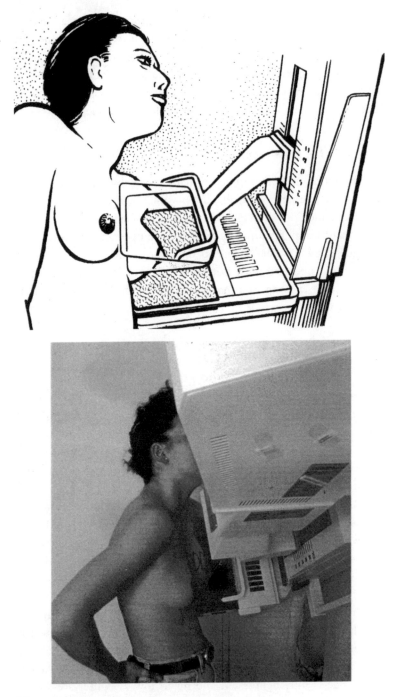

Figure 5.4 A woman having a mammogram.

Cancer tissue in a breast usually gets very small spots of calcium in it. Calcium is the mineral in bone that cannot be penetrated by X-rays and so it makes bones look white on X-rays. A local collection of small spots of calcium (called microcalcification) is usual in most breast cancers, so a local collection of white spots on the mammogram may indicate the presence of a small cancer at that site in the breast, even though often no lump can be felt.

As the doses of X-rays used in mammography are very small, in most cases they do no harm provided they are not repeated too frequently. A mammogram every second year or even once a year is considered quite safe for women over 50. For younger women

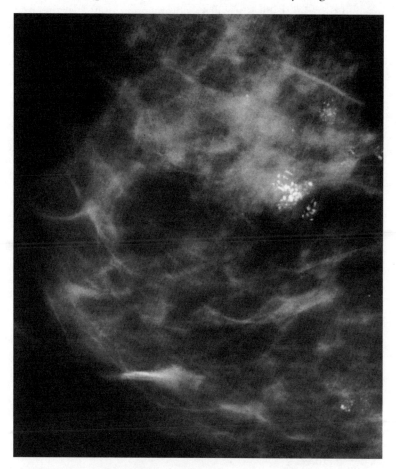

Figure 5.5 The collection of tiny white spots showing in this mammogram indicates the presence of a breast cancer.

who are still ovulating and especially if they may become pregnant, frequent X-rays are not recommended. X-rays, including mammograms, are best avoided, especially during the early stages of pregnancy because early developing foetal tissues may be affected by even very small doses of X-rays. Ultrasound studies may be used in these circumstances as they are quite harmless, even in pregnancy.

Women should be aware that mammography can be uncomfortable. This is because pressure is exerted on the breasts as they are held between two plates. Most women do not find this a major discomfort, but some women do find it uncomfortable and are pleased that the study is usually recommended only every second year.

Mammogram studies are not perfect and occasionally it may not be possible to see a very early cancer. However, most early cancers are detected and quite often they can be detected or a suspicion aroused before even an experienced specialist can feel any abnormality with examining fingers.

Ultrasound

Ultrasound is a study based on the principle of sound waves bouncing back to a recorder from underlying tissues. The degree to which the sound waves bounce back depends on the nature or qualities of the underlying tissues. The principle is similar to that used by fishing crews to detect schools of fish or oceanographers to measure the depth of the ocean floor. Dolphins use a similar system with echoes from their 'clicks' and 'whistles' to locate the schools of fish they feed on.

Ultrasound studies cause no pain, harm or discomfort to the patient. The patient simply lies on her back for possibly a half hour or so and a small metal instrument is moved over the area being examined. The returning sound waves record images on a television screen for the operator to detect any abnormality, and 'pictures' are recorded on a graph paper as something like distorted X-ray pictures.

Ultrasound breast studies are often used in younger women as they do not risk damage to the ovaries or any possible pregnancy, and because they often show the tissues in the firm breasts of young women better than mammograms or other tests.

Experts in the field are needed to interpret the findings of ultrasound studies accurately. Ultrasound is not usually regarded as a screening test but it can help to determine the nature of a lump felt in the breast. They are not a reliable way to tell the difference between a cancer lump and other solid lumps, but they are especially helpful in detecting cysts or other fluid-filled lesions. This is because the echo from a hollow, fluid-filled cyst is different from the echo from a solid lump or cancer.

Detection of 'in situ' cancer

A mammogram will often show that a lump is or is not likely to be cancer, but it is not conclusive on its own. It is not until cancer cells are seen in a specimen of tissue examined under a microscope that a diagnosis of cancer can be certain.

With increasing sensitivity and experience with mammography, increased numbers of early cancers are being detected. An increasing proportion of these early cancers are at a stage described as 'in situ'. In situ carcinoma is at a pre-invasive stage. This means that early malignant features are present in some cells, but the cancer cells are showing no evidence of growing into surrounding tissues and almost certainly have not spread further than the local area where they arose.

Adequate removal of the cancer at this 'in situ' stage will cure the cancer. There will be no need to remove the whole breast, local lymph nodes in the armpit or any other tissue unless another cancer develops in that breast.

Invasive cancer

A cancer that has reached a more dangerous stage is described as 'invasive cancer'. An invasive cancer has more aggressive cells that are likely to penetrate into and damage surrounding tissues. The aggressive cells may also break away from their original mass and invade blood vessels, lymph vessels or other channels or spaces from where they are carried to different organs or tissues. Like seeds of a weed in a garden, they can establish new colonies of 'secondary' cancers that damage other parts of the body. The more anaplastic or abnormal the cells appear under the microscope, the more likely it is that they will behave in this aggressive and dangerous fashion and the more rapidly and more widely they are likely to spread.

Differential diagnosis

The presence of a lump and some other features often seen in breast cancer can also be found in non-malignant conditions so that it is important for the doctor to consider all possibilities before making a diagnosis. This consideration of possibilities is known as 'differential diagnosis'. The symptoms of different types of breast cancer and the more common conditions that may be mistaken for breast cancer are outlined below.

Breast lumps

Single breast lumps and lumpy breasts are common in women of Western countries. Most of these lumps are not cancer. A single breast lump is more likely to be a cancer than is a generalised lumpy breast. In women under 50, a small breast lump may be a cancer, but more often it is caused by something that is not cancer. In women over the age of 50, a single breast lump occurring for the first time is likely to be a cancer.

Although most breast cancers are first seen in women over the age of 50 with a peak incidence at about 60 or 65 years, breast cancer can occur in women of any age. It is rarely seen in teenagers or women under 30 and is also not often found for the first time in women over 90 years of age, but cases have been reported at both extremes of age. This means that any breast lump in a woman of any age must be considered seriously in case it is cancer. Other lumps can easily be confused with cancer, and because delay in diagnosis and treatment of cancer can have serious consequences it is vital to be sure of the exact, correct diagnosis without delay.

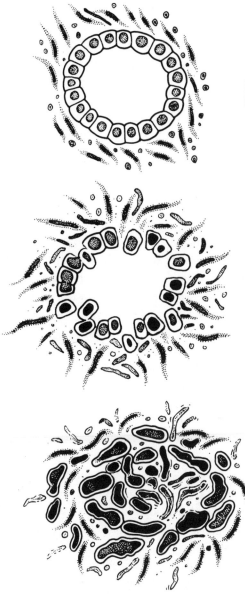

Normal
Breast Tissue

Breast Cancer
"In situ"

Infiltrating
Breast Cancer

Figure 5.6 (a, top) Normal breast tissue. The cells lining the hollow duct are even in size and arranged in an orderly way. (b, centre) Non-invasive 'in situ' breast cancer. A few abnormal-looking cells are disrupting the duct lining. (c, bottom) 'Invasive' or infiltrating breast cancer. The duct has disappeared and the cells no longer resemble normal breast tissue.

Examination by an experienced doctor, mammograms, and sometimes an ultrasound are all important. However, the final diagnosis will depend on taking a biopsy or sample of cells from the suspicious area of the breast, and having an expert pathologist examine the specimen. Different types of biopsy are discussed later in this chapter.

Case report 1 (page 57) illustrates a common scenario for women concerned about a breast lump. As with Mary, in younger women the condition most often is found not to be cancer.

Adenoma, fibroma or fibroadenoma

A painless breast lump in a teenager or young woman is more likely to be caused by a benign fibroma, adenoma or fibroadenoma (see pages 13–14). These are usually felt as a hard round or oval lump that tends to move easily under the fingers when the breast is examined. This is why they are sometimes called a 'breast mouse'. These lumps are not malignant and not prone to become malignant. However, if such a lump is present it is usually better to have it removed by a surgeon to be sure what it is and so that it cannot cause trouble or be confused with cancer later. In any case most women do not like having a lump of any kind in a breast.

Fibrocystic disease

A lump in a breast of a woman in her late thirties or forties is more likely to be a lump or a cyst associated with the condition called *fibrocystic disease*. These lumps are due to hormonal changes affecting the breast, and are associated with breast changes over years of the menstrual cycle. Because a variety of cystic or solid lumpy changes in the breasts can occur with this condition, it has been called by a number of different names over the years. These include *fibroadenosis cystica*, *hormonal mastopathy*, *benign mammary dysplasia* and *chronic mastitis*. These lumps are sometimes painful or tender, especially in the days just before menstruation when they often become more prominent. There are sometimes several lumps in a breast, some bigger than others, and both breasts are likely to be affected, but sometimes a distinct lump is found in one breast only. The condition is more likely to be thought to be cancer when only one lump is felt, especially if it is a painless lump. Lumps due to fibrocystic disease usually develop for the first time during the years of menstruation. They often start to subside after the menopause but they may still be present for some years after the menopause.

The most important aspect of this condition is to make sure that cancer is not present. This is done either by removing a single lump, or by needle biopsy. A breast with lots of small lumps should be kept under regular observation by a doctor. If one or two lumps stand out as being larger, firmer or otherwise different from the others then they should be biopsied. If a new or different or significantly larger lump develops in a generally lumpy breast, it should be biopsied.

If the condition is painful and troublesome there are several possible treatments that can be tried. Some women will respond well to one form of treatment and other women will often respond better to a different treatment, but no one treatment can be relied upon to help all women with lumpy breasts. The treatments range from extra vitamins (especially the B group of vitamins), to diuretics to increase fluid loss by the kidneys, especially at premenstrual times when the breasts may be painful and swollen, simple pain-relieving drugs, or sometimes small doses of hormones. Surgical removal of painful swellings may be the best treatment in bad cases. The natural plant hormones (phytoestrogens), taken daily in tablet form, have recently been found to give a lot of women relief.

Cysts

A cyst in the breast can also sometimes feel like a breast cancer. Although cysts are most often part of the condition known as fibrocystic disease, sometimes a single cyst is present from a number of other causes. The most common is a 'retention cyst'. This is a cyst due to blockage of one of the milk ducts in the breast. If this occurs in association with a pregnancy or breast-feeding it is likely to contain milky fluid and its diagnosis may be fairly obvious, especially if there has been some breast infection during the days of breast-feeding. Sometimes, however, a retention cyst will develop in a breast without any association of pregnancy or lactation. Ultrasound can usually establish that the lump is a cyst, but diagnosis is usually confirmed by the doctor inserting a needle into the lump and sucking out clear, cloudy or milky fluid. After removal of the fluid the lump should disappear, but if it does not disappear or if it recurs quickly it should be surgically removed.

Lumps following injury

Another type of breast lump can follow an injury to the breast. A localised blood clot called a haematoma may be noticed soon after injury, and there may be bruising. Sometimes the haematoma may not have been noticed at the time of injury. Haematomas may gradually become replaced with a lump of scar tissue in a slow healing process. This can sometimes be found as a hard breast lump called an 'organised haematoma' when the original injury has long since been forgotten. Again a biopsy needs to be taken to make sure that the lump is not a cancer. If the lump is not too big, the best way of doing this may be to remove the whole lump surgically and to have it examined by a pathologist.

Fat necrosis

Another cause of a breast lump is a condition called *fat necrosis*. This type of lump is also likely to follow a previous injury that may or may not have been noticed when it occurred. This lump forms when a lot of local fat cells have been damaged and caused a hard local reaction in the tissues that may feel like a breast cancer. Diagnosis and treatment is similar to that of an organised haematoma: biopsy, and where appropriate surgical removal.

Mastitis or breast abscess

A red inflamed swelling in a breast is not uncommon during pregnancy and especially during the days or months of breast-feeding. This is usually caused by invasion of the milk ducts by one of several types of bacteria (germs). The condition called *acute mastitis of pregnancy* may change to form a local abscess in the breast. It usually responds to a standard treatment of completely emptying the breasts with a milk pump, antibiotics, and sometimes stopping breast-feeding using hormones to stop milk production. A localised red, painful, tender abscess will need to be drained by a surgeon.

However, there is a rare form of breast cancer that can look very much like an inflamed breast or a breast abscess. This can occur in older women or in women who have not had a recent pregnancy, and in these women it is not likely to be confused with an abscess of pregnancy. However, this type of cancer can occasionally occur in women who have had a recent pregnancy or who are pregnant. In such cases it is often not recognised as likely to be cancer. A good rule is that if an inflamed or abscessed breast has not responded to appropriate treatment in two weeks then a biopsy should be taken to make sure that it is not a cancer.

A red nipple or nipple rash

In another form of breast cancer, more often seen in older women, no lump may be felt. In this condition, called *Paget's disease of the nipple*, the nipple looks red as though it had been scraped, causing a 'gravel rash' or a crust (see figure 5.36 on p. 41). Usually only one nipple is affected, whereas if this was a simple rash both nipples would be likely to be affected. This condition is best diagnosed by a surgeon taking a small specimen for a biopsy examination.

Fluid or blood discharge from the nipple

Other nipple problems, such as a discharge of fluid or especially of blood from the nipple, may be due to an underlying cancer, although underlying benign fibrocystic disease, or an underlying benign papilloma in a breast duct, are more likely. If underlying fibrocystic disease is the only abnormality found it will need to be treated as previously described. A papilloma will need to be removed surgically and examined under the microscope to be sure that no cancer cells are present.

Other types of breast lumps and tumours

The breast is also occasionally the site of one of the variety of other lumps that can occur in almost any other tissue of the body.

Sometimes a lipoma or fibroma or other benign lump or cyst will be present in or under the skin covering the breast. Similar benign tumours or tumours of muscle, blood vessels or nerves sometimes occur in, under or near the breast. Any of these tumours can occasionally occur in a malignant (cancerous) form as some type of *sarcoma*. However, sarcomas in or close to the breast are rare. When they do occur the diagnosis must be confirmed by biopsy. Such a sarcoma requires the same treatment as a sarcoma in any other part of the body.

A problem not in the breast

An abnormal finding or a health problem not in the breast can sometimes be caused by secondary breast cancer. In these cases, if the patient was known to have previously had a breast cancer it is usually not difficult to relate the new problem to the previous cancer. If a woman who has previously been treated for breast cancer develops a lump under the skin, an enlarged lymph node, a shadow seen in a chest X-ray, a lump in the liver, bone pain or a deposit of tumour in a bone, or evidence of a tumour in the brain, the medical team will be alerted to the possibility that the new problem might be caused by a secondary deposit from breast cancer. Investigations will be made to confirm or deny this suspicion, the most important being a tissue biopsy. If, however, one of these problems arises without any other explanation, the possibility that the woman has a previously undetected breast cancer must be considered. A biopsy of the suspicious tissue will help resolve the diagnosis. If cancer cells are found that are of a type consistent with breast cancer, then further breast studies are required. This is not a common problem, but when it does arise the most common finding is enlarged lymph nodes in an armpit that may be due to a previously unrecognised breast cancer.

Tissue biopsies

No matter how compelling the evidence from mammogram or ultrasound, or from other suspicious features, a lump cannot be assumed to be cancer until cancer cells have been seen. It is therefore essential to have a biopsy for microscopic examination of cells to be sure that the cells are cancer cells. Non-malignant lumps can sometimes look very like cancer, even in mammograms, so it is essential to be sure. By the same token a breast lump cannot be assumed not to be a cancer until the type of cells responsible for the lump have been clearly identified.

There are several ways of taking a specimen of cells for biopsy or microscopic examination. If the patient is in a clinic, the quickest, most convenient and simplest method may be to use a needle and syringe to aspirate (suck out) some cells from the lump. The needle is simply inserted into the lump and a sample of cells is sucked into a syringe containing a special preservative fluid. This is a relatively painless procedure, and a local anaesthetic may or may not be needed. The specimen of cells obtained is sent to an expert pathologist (known as a cytologist) for preparation and microscopic examination.

If a sufficient specimen of cells cannot be obtained by aspiration, a number of other small cutting instruments exist that can be inserted into the lump to take a small 'core' of tissue from the lump. This 'core biopsy' can usually be carried out using only a local anaesthetic, but sometimes a general anaesthetic is preferred for the patient's acceptability and comfort.

Occasionally neither aspiration cytology alone nor 'core' biopsy alone is totally reliable in establishing a diagnosis. In doubtful cases it is sometimes helpful to use both in the same patient.

Sometimes it is essential for the doctor to have a larger or more representative specimen of the lump for examination, especially if there is some doubt about the type of cells seen under the microscope. A small operation may be required for the surgeon to cut out a small piece of tissue for examination or, if the lump is small, occasionally the whole lump is removed and sent for microscopic examination.

If a lump felt in a breast is found to be cancer and mammograms were not performed, it may be important to have mammograms of the other breast to try to be sure that it is clear of cancer before final treatment is carried out.

Image guided needle biopsy

If a lump cannot be felt but mammograms have suggested that a certain area in a breast has features that look like breast cancer, it is sometimes necessary to use X-ray screening to help guide a needle into the suspected area to take a biopsy of the suspect tissue.

Frozen-section examination

Occasionally if a pre-operative biopsy leaves some doubt as to whether a breast lump is a cancer and for one reason or another it is better for the patient to have an operation for cure without delay, the patient can be prepared for the operation under a general anaesthetic. But before a major operation, like removal of the breast, is carried out, a small piece of the lump is taken and sent to a special laboratory for 'frozen-section' examination. In this examination the specialist pathologist immediately freezes the specimen to make it hard so that it can be sliced finely and stained for immediate microscopic examination. The pathologist can then give a report on the nature of the lump while the surgical team is preparing for whatever operation the patient may need. The different possibilities will have been discussed with the patient before the operation so that the patient's preferred choice and acceptance of treatment will be known by the surgical team.

Frozen-section biopsies for breast lumps were once a common procedure, but they are not commonly used now that pre-operative needle or core biopsies have become more and more reliable.

Hormone receptor testing

If a tissue biopsy reveals cancer, it is important to determine the cancer's sensitivity to different hormones. These hormone receptor studies are made by the pathology team on the specimen sent for biopsy examination. The information they give about the cancer's sensitivity to hormones may be valuable in deciding the most appropriate treatment for that particular cancer. These studies are now practised as a routine in all good pathology laboratories, especially on excised pieces of biopsy tissue, but also on core biopsy tissue. Nowadays hormone receptor studies can often be made with good aspiration cytology specimens.

Case report 1: *Mary, aged 44*

Mary is a teacher, married with two children. Mary had become aware of increasing premenstrual breast discomfort over several months but had not had previous mammograms. One day while having her morning shower, she noticed a lump in the right breast between the nipple and the outer edge of the breast. She consulted her doctor, who also felt the lump and noted that it was a little tender. The doctor noticed a little generalised nodularity or lumpiness throughout that breast, but the lump Mary had found was quite distinct. The doctor immediately arranged for Mary to have mammogram X-rays and to see a specialist surgeon.

The mammogram report said that there were some increased markings in both breasts, with a dense collection of fibrous tissue in the right breast just to one side of the nipple. There was nothing specific to suggest cancer. The report advised that fibrocystic disease was the likely diagnosis but recommended a biopsy to be sure.

The specialist surgeon agreed with the findings of his colleagues and arranged for Mary to have a needle aspiration cytology biopsy of the breast lump.

The needle biopsy was performed next day with Mary as an outpatient. The lump was smaller after some fluid had been drawn off, and the report stated that no cancer cells could be found. The cells seen were consistent with a diagnosis of fibrocystic disease.

Mary was shown how to do regular self-examination of her breasts and advised to do this in the bath on a monthly basis after completion of menstruation. She was given B complex vitamins to take daily, and was advised to take one phytoestrogen tablet daily. She was also advised to see her family doctor in two months, or sooner if she had any new worry, and to make an appointment to see the specialist surgeon again in four months and then on an annual basis. She would have a repeat mammogram in one year and thereafter would have a mammogram every second year unless anything new developed.

Five years later Mary remains well with no new breast lumps. She can still feel a little general nodularity or lumpiness in her breasts, especially before menstruation. For more than four years she continued to menstruate regularly, but her menstruation has recently become less regular with the apparent onset of menopause.

Approaches to treatment

The most common first sign that a woman has breast cancer is when she finds a lump in her breast, although routine screening by mammography is now detecting increasing numbers of early cancers when no lump has been felt in the breasts.

If breast cancer is diagnosed, it is important to discover how early or advanced, and how aggressive, the cancer is, and whether it has spread into nearby lymph nodes or into more distant tissues. Determining this is called 'tumour staging', and until the stage is known it will not be possible to plan the most appropriate treatment.

Staging breast cancer

Pre-invasive (in situ) breast cancer

Many early breast cancers detected by routine screening mammography are at a stage called 'in situ' or 'pre-invasive' cancer (see figure 5.6 on p.49). Cancer cells have developed but they have remained in the same place. Cancer detected at this stage is eminently curable and, provided it is the only part of the breast with any such trouble in it, it is usually treated by surgical removal of that part of the breast. This is usually followed up with radiotherapy 'just in case' there is any more cancer in the breast that needs to be mopped up.

Invasive breast cancer

If a diagnosis of 'invasive' breast cancer has been established, it is important to establish how early or how advanced this cancer is. The cancer cells may have spread a little into nearby breast tissue only, or they may have spread further. The most appropriate treatment depends mainly on the stage of the tumour, but other factors will be taken into account. These include the degree of abnormality (anaplasia) of the cancer cells, and the age and general health of the patient.

Four basic tumour stages are recognised.

Stage I cancer is a small cancer that may have spread a little into nearby breast tissues but is still totally confined to the breast. It has not spread to lymph nodes or other tissues or organs, and has not grown into overlying skin or the underlying muscles of the chest wall.

Stage II cancer can be a localised breast lump (up to about 5 centimetres) that has spread into the nearby lymph nodes in the armpit but has not spread further into distant tissues or organs.

Stage III cancer indicates a larger cancer in the breast that has usually spread into lymph nodes and possibly has become attached to skin or to muscle, or which is attached to tissues around the lymph nodes, but there is no evidence that it has spread into distant tissues or organs.

Stage IV cancer is a cancer that has spread already, with secondaries in tissues or organs away from the breast.

Investigations

Before any major operation is carried out in an attempt to cure breast cancer, it is essential to be as sure as is possible that the cancer is confined to the breast only and has not spread anywhere else, other than possibly into lymph nodes in the nearby armpit. The cancer should then be curable by removing part of or the whole of the breast, possibly with nearby lymph nodes from the armpit.

A chest X-ray and 'full blood count' will help determine the general health of the patient and her fitness for treatment. Occasionally they may show evidence of cancer spread. For example, the

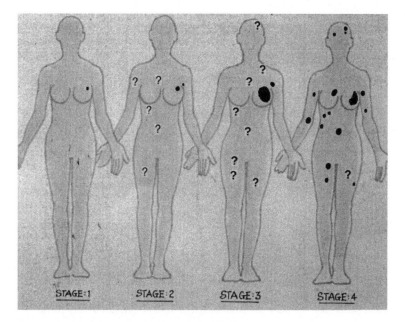

Figure 6.1 The four 'stages' of breast cancer.

blood studies may show evidence of anaemia, and this could be due to bone secondaries (metastases) destroying the blood-forming cells in bone marrow. The other tests usually carried out before operation for breast cancer are also more or less routine tests for general health conducted before any major operation on any part of the body. These tests, called *liver function tests* and *serum electro-lyte*, are blood tests to detect any evidence of liver disturbance and to confirm the general health and fitness for operation of the patient.

For people with an advanced cancer or cancer associated with bone pain, *isotope bone scans* may be needed to show any evidence of bone metastases. The isotope scans are something like special X-rays, and require a very small amount of a special radioactive isotope material to be injected into a vein before the scanning procedure. The scanning procedure is quite painless. Isotope scans will usually indicate possible metastases in bones before they can be seen in X-rays, but X-rays should also be taken for more pre-cise and more detailed information of metastatic bone damage. Breast cancer metastases in bones may show up as pale areas of partly destroyed bone, or occasionally as dense white, calcified (sclerotic) areas in the bone. Chest X-rays may show evidence of metastases in the lungs, in lymph nodes in the chest, or even in the ribs.

Women with large or advanced cancers may also require a type of very specialised X-ray called a CT scan, not only to show the size and extent of the cancer in the breast region but also to check whether the cancer can be seen to have spread further into distant tissues. CT studies of breast and abdomen may be made especially to look for any possible evidence of cancer spread into the lungs, liver, ovaries or elsewhere.

If a lump is found in some other part of the body, other than in the breast involved, it is sometimes necessary to take a biopsy sample of the lump to know whether the cells in it have come from the breast cancer. Sometimes such biopsies can be carried out as a minor procedure and without a general anaesthetic. However, especially for suspected tumours in such organs as liver, bone or lung, a general anaesthetic may be required.

Nowadays, in a very few highly specialised cancer centres, a new scanning procedure called a PET scan (positron emission tomography) is being studied. As yet this type of scan is not available in most centres. Whether PET scans will prove to have important additional value in breast cancer studies is not yet known. Certainly at this stage PET scanning is important for research and future medical knowledge and progress, but as yet it is not important for patient care.

What treatments are available?

Once a breast cancer has been diagnosed, a decision must be made about most appropriate treatment. The most appropriate treatment will depend especially on the stage of the cancer. Important features to consider include the size of the lump, its position in the breast, its possible attachment to overlying skin or underlying muscles, involvement of nearby (armpit) lymph nodes, and any evidence of spread of the cancer to other lymph nodes or other parts of the body. The degree of potential aggressiveness of the cancer cells (anaplasia) will also be a factor. All this information will be taken into account in relation to the age and general health of the patient, any family history of breast cancer or other relevant factors, the patient's social and domestic circumstances, best treatment facilities available, and follow-up and continuing care facilities available.

The patient's help in choice of treatment

A most important factor is the patient's personal attitude to the cancer and to her breasts. Her personal attitude and needs are often very relevant to choice of treatment. For example, if a choice is to be made between two treatments that are likely to give equally satisfactory results then these should be discussed with the patient to allow her personal needs and wishes to be taken into consideration. The treatment team or surgeon should advise but should not try to forcefully persuade the patient to accept a particular treatment procedure unless there is clear evidence that better overall results are likely to be achieved by that procedure.

An example of this possible conflict in choice of treatment is in treatment of a relatively small and apparently localised stage I breast cancer. A decision must be made as to whether the whole breast should be removed or whether to carry out a breast-saving procedure. In this procedure, only that part of the breast containing the cancer is removed and the remaining breast tissue is treated with radiotherapy. Evidence suggests that there is no significant difference as far as long-term cure is concerned. Surgeons generally assume that it is preferable to save most of the breast, and this is probably the case for most patients. There are some women, however, who would feel more comfortable if a breast with a cancer in it was totally removed; otherwise they would continue to be very concerned about the possibility of further trouble developing in any part of the breast left behind. Even though the surgeon might be convinced that this is not a realistic cause for concern, the options should be clearly discussed with the patient, and the patient's needs and wishes should be taken into account. Ultimately the choice of treatment must be the patient's.

Surgical treatment

Surgery can be used in treatment of breast cancer with one or more of the following objectives:

- To establish a diagnosis by tissue biopsy, that is to establish that a cancer is present (discussed above). Occasionally a biopsy may also be needed to establish whether any lump or other trouble away from the breast is due to a metastasis (secondary).
- To remove the cancer totally and achieve a cure, either by operation alone, or in combination with radiotherapy or other forms of treatment (chapters 7 and 8).
- To relieve symptoms of pain or discomfort if the cancer is not curable, or to attend troubles caused by metastases (chapter 9).
- To reconstruct a breast (chapter 10).

Pre-admission advice

If an operation is planned the surgeon will advise the patient about aspects of the procedure with which she may not be familiar. The surgeon will explain that the operation will be performed under a general anaesthetic and she will wake up in a hospital ward bed. She will feel some pain in the breast region and will be given pain-relieving injections. She will have a dressing on her wound and probably a small drain tube from the wound to a bottle beside the bed. She will have a drip of fluid running into a vein in her arm. She will not want to move the arm much for a day or two, but then will be encouraged to exercise the arm gently. She will usually be able to walk the day after the operation and usually may expect to go home in from three to eight days.

Hospital admission

Until recently the patient was usually admitted to hospital on the day before the operation was planned, but it is now common practice for the patient to be admitted on the day operation is to be carried out. There in the ward she will meet the various members of the treatment team and especially the resident doctors and nursing team who will be caring for her. Any necessary tests like blood count, chest X-ray, liver function tests and other blood tests like serum electrolytes are commonly completed before admission on an outpatient basis.

The patient will be admitted by a member of the nursing team. A medical admission with details of her health problems will be taken by a doctor, who will also carry out a general examination. If the patient has not previously been examined by the anaesthetist, she will be examined by the anaesthetist before the operation. These people will be able to answer her questions about the procedure or help her with any other problems with which she is not familiar.

The patient will have been advised to eat and drink freely until the evening before operation, but thereafter not to eat or drink for 8 or 10 hours before the time scheduled for operation as this could cause vomiting during the anaesthetic. She will usually have been given a calming or tranquillising tablet to ensure a good rest on the night before operation. An hour or so before operation she will be given a 'premedication' injection as a calming agent and to prepare her for the anaesthetic.

Radiotherapy, hormone therapy and chemotherapy

Current treatments with radiotherapy, hormone therapy or chemotherapy are unlikely to achieve a cure when used alone, but when used in combination with surgery these treatments can make a cure more certain. In some cases they can be used in conjunction with surgery to achieve a cure when cure by surgery alone is unlikely. They can also be used to relieve symptoms and pain from cancer metastases when cure is unlikely.

All these approaches and combinations of approaches are discussed in the following chapters.

Stage I breast cancer

Stage I breast cancer is a cancer that is small and has been diagnosed in its early stage, before it has spread outside the breast. If the patient is young enough and fit enough to have an operation, consideration should be given either to carrying out total removal of the breast (total mastectomy) or, in the case of a small lump, removal of that section of the breast containing the cancer (partial mastectomy or segmentectomy) followed by radiotherapy to the breast. Another option offered by some surgeons is simply to remove the lump (lumpectomy) and to follow this with radiotherapy to the breast. Most studies suggest that it is safer to remove a little more than just the lump, but whatever operation is used, radiotherapy is recommended in case some cancer cells have been left behind in the breast. For stage I breast cancer any one of these three procedures is very likely to achieve a cure—the cure rate should be more than 80 per cent with any of these three treatment procedures.

Case reports 2 and 3 are examples of two women who received appropriate surgical treatment for stage I breast cancer.

Regular mammogram studies now commonly used in cancer screening clinics are detecting increasing numbers of pre-invasive 'in situ' cancers. Provided there is only one such area in a breast, adequate removal of that area may be all that is needed to cure that cancer. However, remaining breast tissue is usually treated by radiotherapy in case further malignant cells are present. The breast can otherwise be left intact but the woman is kept under regular observation, including further regular mammogram screening studies. For 'in situ' cancer there should be no need to remove axillary (armpit) lymph nodes as these will not have become invaded.

For early 'invasive' cancer, that is cancer that is a little more locally invasive than 'in situ' cancer but still apparently stage I with no lymph node involvement, surgeons have different opinions and different experiences with the three treatment options. For women who are very keen to save their breast, either segmentectomy, partial mastectomy or lumpectomy, all with follow-up irradiation, might be considered appropriate. However, as already discussed, some women do not feel comfortable unless a breast with a cancer in it has been totally removed. They have no wish to retain any part of this breast. If after proper explanation this remains their well considered choice, then a mastectomy would be the most appropriate treatment.

Regardless of the choice of treatment of the breast, if 'invasive' or 'infiltrating' cancer has been diagnosed a decision has to be made about axillary (armpit) lymph nodes. It is important to know whether or not any of these nodes have cancer cells growing in them. If the nodes can be felt to be enlarged and hard or if they appear to be abnormal in ultrasound studies, and a decision has been made to remove them all regardless, there is no need for a 'node sampling' procedure.

Sentinel node sampling

Sentinel node sampling is a recently developed special test that can help the surgeon to find the lymph node or nodes into which tissue fluid from the affected part of the breast drains. If the cancer has spread into the lymph nodes, these are the nodes most likely to contain cancer. These nodes, called the 'sentinel' nodes, are removed for examination in any patient with 'invasive' breast cancer. The theory is that if no cancer is found in the sentinel node or nodes there should be no need to remove any more nodes in the armpit. Although this test is highly reliable for another type of cancer (melanoma of skin), as yet it is not known how reliable this test will be in showing the first evidence of spread of breast cancer. Studies are continuing and more certainty of the value of this test should be known within a year or two of publication of this book. At this stage the test appears to be a good guide as to which nodes should be removed and examined to get the most reliable information about likely the spread of breast cancer.

If cancer is found in one or more sentinel nodes the cancer is a stage II cancer, and there is a risk that it might be in other nodes. All nodes are therefore surgically excised from that armpit.

There are two ways of locating the sentinel nodes. One is by *lymphoscintigraphy* and the other is by the *blue dye test*.

In lymphoscintigraphy, a small dose of a weakly radioactive substance is injected near the cancer site in the breast and a nuclear scanner is used to discover where in the armpit the radioactivity becomes concentrated. This indicates the site of the lymph node or nodes (sentinel nodes) into which fluid from this part of the breast drains. Small tattoo marks are made in the overlying skin to show the surgeon just where these sentinel nodes are when the operation is performed. Lymphoscintigraphy can now also be used to look for possible sentinel nodes in the chest or in the neck. Sentinel nodes in these areas are uncommon, but if they are found ultrasound studies can help find whether lymph nodes in these areas are likely to have cancer in them.

The blue dye test is similar. Instead of the radioactive substance, a small amount of blue dye is injected into the breast near the cancer. The blue dye then travels to the nearest draining lymph nodes, the sentinel nodes. When the surgeon operates a couple of hours later it is easy to find the conspicuous blue lymph nodes that need to be taken out and examined for evidence of any cancer spread.

Axillary node sampling

As yet the reliability of sentinel node biopsy has not been confirmed and the practice of sentinel node biopsy is still not widely performed. In hospitals and clinics where sentinel node biopsy is not performed, most surgeons remove the lymph nodes closest to the breast cancer and have them examined under the microscope. This is called 'axillary node sampling'. If any cancer cells are found in any of the sampled nodes, then all lymph nodes in that armpit are usually removed. If no cancer is found in the lymph nodes closest to the cancer then further removal of lymph nodes is usually not carried out, as it is not likely that the cancer has spread further.

Ultrasound node studies

The use of ultrasound has recently been refined and improved to a degree where, in the hands of experts, ultrasound examination of lymph nodes can give a very good indication as to whether the nodes do or probably do not contain metastatic cancer. Such ultrasound studies can be a very useful guide to the surgeon or to the radiotherapist if abnormal lymph nodes are found in the chest or neck, places not likely to be cured by surgery. If it appears likely that lymph nodes in the lower neck might be involved with cancer they are usually treated with additional radiotherapy. Radiotherapy to treat lymph nodes in the chest is avoided unless absolutely necessary because it poses the risk of radiation damage to important organs in the chest such as the heart or lungs.

Case report 2: *Jean, aged 51*

Jean is a full-time mother of three children, and had passed through the menopause without any problem a year or two before. She had been in the habit of performing regular self-examination of her breasts in the bath after her menstrual period finished, and had maintained the practice. One evening in the bath she felt a small firm lump in the upper outer part of her left breast. Her husband could not feel the lump, but Jean was sufficiently concerned to visit her doctor next day. The doctor could feel the lump, and arranged for Jean to have mammogram X-rays. The mammograms showed a small area of dense tissue in the upper outer part of her left breast. This tissue contained several small spots of calcification that were highly suggestive of a small breast cancer. Jean's doctor arranged a consultation with a specialist surgeon. The surgeon agreed that the findings looked like cancer, and arranged with a pathologist to have a biopsy carried out the same day. A needle was inserted into the lump under a local anaesthetic, and some cells were sucked out into a syringe containing fluid. This material was then examined microscopically. Cancer cells were seen, so the diagnosis of cancer was certain. The surgeon could find no evidence of enlarged lymph nodes in Jean's armpit, and investigations did not show any evidence that the cancer had spread beyond the breast.

The surgeon arranged to discuss the possible plans of treatment with Jean and her husband together. Jean was advised that a sentinel node study by lymphoscintigraphy could help to identify the lymph nodes most at risk of cancer spread, so this was performed. Small tattoo marks were made in the skin directly over the sentinel nodes to guide the surgeon to the position of these nodes during the operation.

Jean was admitted to hospital the next week and operation was carried out on the day after admission. The surgeon did a second test to identify the sentinel nodes. A blue dye was injected near the breast lump two hours before the operation so that when operation was carried out the blue dye would make the sentinel lymph nodes easier to find. The segment of the breast containing the cancer was removed at the operation together with the sentinel lymph nodes that had stained blue. These lymph nodes were otherwise normal, so no further lymph nodes were removed. Later pathology studies confirmed the presence of a small cancer in the section of breast removed but no cancer cells were found in the sentinel lymph nodes.

Jean made a good recovery from the operation. She started shoulder exercises on the day following surgery. The fluid drip in her vein was removed next day, and she began eating solid foods. The wound drain was removed on the fifth day. Jean was allowed home on the sixth day after the operation. She returned to the hospital on the tenth day to have her stitches removed, and sticky paper strips were placed across the wound to support it for a few more days.

A consultation had been made with a radiotherapist, who advised Jean that the breast should be treated by radiotherapy in case any cancer cells remained. Jean agreed, and radiotherapy was commenced three weeks after surgery. Radiotherapy was given on each week day over five weeks.

Three years later Jean remains well. She visits her doctor every three months and sees the surgeon once a year. Further mammograms of both breasts are planned for every second year.

Case report 3: *Liz, aged 36*

Liz was a 36-year-old hairdresser. She was in the twentieth week of her first pregnancy when she noticed a distinct lump in the upper part of her left breast, a little towards the armpit. The lump was just a little tender so her immediate thought was that it was simply a retention cyst related to her pregnancy, but she attended her doctor 'just in case'. Her doctor too thought that, in view of Liz's young age, her pregnancy and the slight tenderness in the lump, it was likely to be a small cyst. No enlarged lymph nodes were detected. However, to help to be sure about the diagnosis, an ultrasound study was arranged for the next day.

The ultrasound showed that the lump was not a cyst but was a solid lump, so a biopsy by needle aspiration was arranged immediately. This examination showed the presence of cancer cells.

Liz wished to continue her pregnancy. After discussion with her husband and her doctor, she decided to have her left breast removed. She was advised that surgery was safest in the middle of her pregnancy (the second trimester) rather than at the beginning or near the end of her pregnancy, so the operation was arranged forthwith.

Lymph nodes closest to the tumour were removed with the breast. The pathology report confirmed that a small cancer was present in the breast but no cancer was found in the lymph nodes.

Liz made a good recovery and sixteen weeks later delivered a normal healthy baby girl, whom she breast-fed with her right breast. She has since undergone reconstruction of a left breast. Her daughter is now eight years old and Liz, her daughter and her husband are all well and happy.

Liz continues to have regular checks with her doctors, including ultrasounds and mammograms of her right breast.

8

Stage II breast cancer

If the cancer is relatively small in the breast but there is evidence that it has spread into lymph nodes in the armpit, but no further, it is classified as stage II cancer.

There are several surgical options of treatment for stage II breast cancer. This is because no one treatment has been shown to achieve better results than other treatment options in all circumstances.

The treatment that has been carried out most over the years is called radical mastectomy. This means the breast is removed totally, together with all lymph nodes from the nearby armpit, all in one continuous block of tissue. This procedure is called a radical block dissection. Worldwide this may still be the most common procedure used to treat stage II breast cancer. However, for small breast lumps, studies have shown that comparable long-term cure rates can be achieved with partial mastectomy or segmentectomy accompanied by removal of the lymph nodes and followed up by radiotherapy. This operation, in which most of the breast is left in place, is called breast conserving or breast salvage surgery. Worldwide experience has now shown that in 80 per cent of women with breast cancer a breast conserving operation followed by radiotherapy will give equally good long-term results without need to remove the whole breast. In about 20 per cent of women the cancer is of such a size or in such a position that total removal of the breast is needed.

If lymph nodes in the armpit are found to have cancer in them there is a risk that the cancer may have spread further, even if X-rays, scans and other tests have not been able to detect it in other tissues. The long-term cure rates for these women are improved if they are given follow-up treatment, called adjuvant treatment, either with chemotherapy (usually for younger fitter women) or hormone treatment (usually for older women). With adjuvant treatment, long-term (10 years) cure rates for women with stage II breast cancer have been found to be improved by at least 10 per cent and possibly more. Adjuvant treatment is discussed further on pages 96–7.

Case report 4 describes the experiences of a woman whose stage II breast cancer was managed using surgery, radiotherapy and chemotherapy. Case report 5 is an example of a woman with a stage II breast cancer that was treated using surgery, radiotherapy and tamoxifen.

Case report 4: *Susan, aged 58*

Susan was a 58-year-old business executive. She had always been single, and had no children or other close family. While she was being examined by her doctor for a general health check, the doctor found a thickened lumpy mass in the upper outer part of her left breast. The mass was about three centimetres in diameter but was movable. Susan had not been aware of any breast trouble.

The doctor arranged mammography and biopsy by aspiration cytology, and both reports indicated a diagnosis of cancer. The doctor arranged a consultation with a specialist surgeon who then arranged several tests, including a chest X-ray, blood count, blood typing and blood biochemistry.

The surgeon could feel two hard enlarged lymph nodes in the left armpit. In discussing possible methods of treatment with Susan, the surgeon recommended that the quadrant of the breast containing the cancer should be removed together with the lymph nodes in the left armpit. The surgeon advised Susan to consult a radiotherapist for advice and treatment of the remaining breast tissue and possibly the armpit region, in case any cancer cells were left behind after surgery. A date for Susan's hospital admission was arranged and the consultation with the radiotherapist organised.

The radiotherapist agreed with the treatment plan proposed by the surgeon.

The operation was carried out without any significant problem. After the operation Susan woke to find that she had a painful wound region, a small drain from under the wound dressings was draining into a bottle on the side of the bed, and a drip of fluid was running into a vein in her arm. She was allowed out of bed the next day and encouraged to walk a little more each day. Susan was also encouraged to move her left arm gently a little more each day to get a gradual return of the full range of shoulder movement. She was allowed to drink some fluids on the day following the operation and commenced a little soft food on the next day. On the fourth day she was back on a normal diet. The drip in her arm was removed after 24 hours but the wound drainage tube was left for five days until drainage had stopped. She was allowed home after seven days. She revisited the surgeon on the tenth day after operation, and the stitches were removed and replaced by sticky tapes.

Three weeks after leaving hospital her radiotherapy was commenced.

As four of the 25 lymph nodes taken from the armpit were found to contain cancer cells, an appointment was made for Susan to be seen by a specialist medical oncologist. The oncologist arranged for a program of chemotherapy to be commenced two weeks after the course of radiotherapy had been completed.

Susan lost her hair during the chemotherapy treatment and arranged to wear a wig that matched her original hair. After the course of chemotherapy was finished, Susan's hair grew again, rather thicker and a little darker than her original hair. She returned to her business and has since remained well. She had regular medical checks, at first three monthly then six monthly, and now, after five years, has medical checks on an annual basis. She also has an annual mammogram of both breasts.

Susan joined a breast cancer support group. At first she got a lot of support and advice from the group, and now she is able to give advice, help and support to other women facing breast cancer problems.

Case report 5: *Peggy, aged 69*

Peggy is a retired nurse. She is the mother of a grown-up family of five, and her husband had died six years previously. When having her daily bath Peggy noticed a lump in her right breast. She visited her doctor immediately. The doctor also felt the lump, and referred her to a surgeon who specialised in treatment of breast cancer. The surgeon examined the breast lump, but also felt enlarged lymph nodes in the right armpit. Aspiration cytology (biopsy with a needle) was arranged and cancer in the breast lump was confirmed. Peggy's chest X-ray and blood count were normal. There was no evidence of cancer spread beyond the lymph nodes in the armpit, so arrangements were made for Peggy to be admitted to hospital for surgery the next week.

The surgeon discussed treatment options and recommended a partial removal of the breast. Peggy said that she would prefer to have the breast totally removed with removal of all lymph nodes from the armpit, even though this was not the surgeon's recommendation. The surgeon carried out her wish.

The operation was uneventful. Peggy was encouraged to move her arm and shoulder gently on the first day after the operation, when she was also encouraged to get out of bed and walk a little and take some fluids by mouth. She was given a little soft food to eat next day when the drip of fluid into a vein in her arm was removed. She could then exercise and walk a little more and was eating and drinking as she wished on the third day. The drainage tube was removed from her wound on the seventh day after surgery, and next day Peggy was allowed home to the care of her daughter. She was advised to continue her gentle arm and shoulder exercises. The wound had been closed with metal clips and all clips were removed on the twelfth day. Small adhesive paper strips were placed across the wound to be left for a few days to give the wound support after the clips were removed.

Six of the 29 lymph nodes removed were found to contain cancer, so Peggy was seen by a medical oncologist. Peggy expressed a wish not to have chemotherapy as in her nursing experience she had seen many cases of complete hair loss and other unpleasant side-effects, especially in older women. The medical oncologist instead recommended follow-up hormone treatment with tamoxifen daily for two years. Peggy joined a breast cancer support club where she was able both to receive and to give useful advice.

Peggy is very active physically and socially. She wears a prosthesis in her bra and was offered breast reconstruction surgery but declined. She has attended her doctor regularly and her specialist twice yearly and remains well three years later.

(9)

Stage III and stage IV breast cancer

Stage III breast cancer

A stage III breast cancer will have one or more of the following features:
- A large tumour lump in the breast (5 centimetres or more across).
- The lump is attached to the chest muscle under the breast, or the lump is attached to and possibly growing through the skin over it.
- Enlarged lymph nodes in the armpit are attached to other tissues in the armpit, so that the nodes cannot be easily moved.
- No evidence is found of cancer spread to more distant tissues or organs such as lung, liver or bone.

It is unlikely that a stage III cancer could be totally removed by surgery alone. There is a risk of some cancer cells being left behind and growing again in the operation wound, so for this stage of cancer it is usually better not to use major surgery as the first treatment. It is usually better to use non-surgical treatments first, often radiotherapy or chemotherapy or hormone treatment, or two or more of these in combination. These treatments will usually make the cancer smaller and control it for a long time; very occasionally they even appear to cure it.

With stage III breast cancer, even if the initial treatment appears to be successful, there is a considerable risk that the cancer will return in the breast region. There is also a risk that although it was thought to be a stage III breast cancer, sooner or later secondary cancer will be found in other tissues, such as in lymph nodes in other parts of the body, the lungs, the liver, the ovaries, or in bones. Such secondaries show that the cancer was not really stage III when detected but was stage IV and clearly not curable by surgery. Fortunately most breast cancers are detected and treated when they are much smaller (stage I or stage II) and at a likely curable stage.

Sometimes a true stage III cancer, that is a big cancer with no secondaries other than possibly in the armpit lymph nodes, can be made much smaller with chemotherapy or with radiotherapy or with both chemotherapy and radiotherapy. If the cancer has not already spread it can sometimes be reduced in size so that it can be removed surgically with a good chance of cure. This technique of combined treatment is discussed in later chapters.

Stage IV breast cancer

Occasionally a breast cancer is not detected until it can already be found to have spread into other parts of the body. This is therefore a stage IV cancer and it is clearly not curable by operating on the breast alone. Evidence of spread to other places is usually con-firmed in bone scans, bone X-rays, chest X-rays, liver scans or CT scans. As yet it is not certain whether the new, somewhat experi-mental, techniques of PET scanning will help significantly in detecting the spread of the cancer beyond the breast.

A stage IV breast cancer may spread to virtually any part of the body, but lungs, bones, liver, the ovaries, other lymph nodes and lumps under the skin anywhere are among the most common secondary sites.

Sometimes a lump is found in tissue some distance from the breasts in a woman who was not known to have had a breast cancer or was treated for breast cancer some years previously. Such a lump can be biopsied to discover exactly what it is. If it is found to be a cancer, the pathologist can usually advise what sort of cancer it is and where it is likely to have come from. It is rare that such a lump is found to be a metastatic breast cancer in a woman who was not aware of any trouble in her breasts, but it can happen.

In spite of there being evidence of more widespread cancer, it is sometimes still a good thing to remove the breast if a stage IV cancer in the breast is relatively small and can be removed surgically. This prevents the risk of the cancer becoming very big and possibly growing through the skin, causing pain and discomfort. If the cancer in the breast is large and causing discomfort and other symptoms it can often be made smaller and even removed using 'combined' or 'integrated' treatment, but as there is still cancer in other places the whole cancer disease will not have been cured.

Inflammatory breast cancer

Most breast cancers are felt as painless, non-tender lumps in the breast, but there is an uncommon type of breast cancer in which an area of the breast or even the whole breast appears to be red and inflamed (see figure 9.1). The condition looks very like a breast with an abscess in it and if it occurs at about the time of a pregnancy or soon after a pregnancy it may be assumed to be an infection and the diagnosis of cancer may be missed. If a breast infection does not respond to appropriate treatment, including antibiotics, within a week or two, then the possibility of there being an inflammatory breast cancer must be considered and investigated. Investigations should include a biopsy.

Inflammatory cancer is an aggressive form of breast cancer. It is usually at least a stage III cancer when detected and often has spread further to become a stage IV cancer. Intensive treatment usually requires chemotherapy, radiotherapy and possibly follow-up surgical mastectomy.

Surgery to relieve symptoms

Sometimes in stage IV breast cancer there is a real risk that the cancer in the breast will grow larger, possibly breaking through the skin and causing ulceration, discomfort and pain. Even though a stage IV cancer cannot be cured by surgery, it is often better to

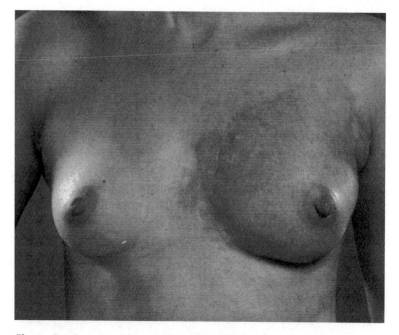

Figure 9.1 Breasts with an 'inflammatory' cancer in the left breast.

remove the breast to give the patient relief of pain or discomfort. This is usually best done after the cancer is first made smaller with chemotherapy or radiotherapy or both.

Sometimes surgery can also be helpful in removing a secondary cancer lump in another part of the body or in fixing a bone that is broken or weakened because of a secondary cancer in it. Even though the operation will not cure the disease, it will often relieve symptoms or prevent further troubles from developing in that part of the body.

(10)

Breast reconstruction surgery

The breast forms an important part of physical and sexual identity for most women. As such there is a wide variety of attitudes towards possible loss of a breast. The extremes range from not wanting to lose a breast at almost any cost, to not wanting to retain any part of a breast that has had a cancer in it.

To a minority of women, more likely older women, a breast may be little more than an unnecessary body appendage, and a breast with a cancer in it is best removed and hopefully forgotten. To others, and especially to younger women, a breast is a very important component of her femininity, sexual completeness and attractiveness. For these women, if a mastectomy is carried out the question of a surgical breast reconstruction will arise.

There are different types of breast reconstruction that may or may not be suitable for the individual patient's needs. The different options should be considered by the patient, as well as by the surgeon and other members of the treatment team who are in a position to contribute to the decision-making in the best interests of the patient's appearance and welfare.

Many women who have had a breast totally removed will be satisfied to have a comfortable prosthesis or 'padding' to fill the empty bra cup and restore external appearance to normal. Some sort of filling is especially necessary for women with a remaining large breast on the other side; otherwise not only does their appearance look unbalanced but their clothes do not fit comfortably and well. All breast clinics have someone, often a trained nurse or an experienced social worker, who is best able to advise on the most suitable appliance to use, and there are several companies that are experienced in fitting women with a very suitable prosthesis for the otherwise empty bra cup.

Breast reconstruction with an implant or with living tissue requires at least one surgical operation. It is not suitable for every patient after mastectomy, but for many women breast reconstruction may not only be appropriate but possibly very desirable for their well being. An expert reconstructive or plastic surgeon must be involved with other members of the treatment team in the choice of reconstructive procedures and their timing. Some surgeons are prepared to reconstruct a new breast at the time of mastectomy in some suitable patients. Until recently most surgeons preferred to wait at least two years after the mastectomy operation until they could feel comfortable that there was little risk of cancer recurring in the breast region. However, it has now been shown that this wait is not necessary. Results are equally good if breast reconstruction is carried out without delay.

The simplest and most readily available reconstructive procedure is a breast implant, in which a plastic prosthesis is placed under the skin of the breast region. A good match in size is easy to arrange and a match in shape is usually quite good, but the soft texture of a normal breast is not so well matched. Nor is there a nipple replacement. Early plastic implants consisted of a colourless or white plastic material filled with a silicone gel. Occasionally such an implant will rupture or leak the silicone gel into surrounding tissues. Such a leak of gel has occasionally caused some tissue damage, but more often it appeared to cause a great deal of anxiety. Concern about silicone implants has been a source of much litigation by women affected or greatly worried by them. Nowadays the plastic prosthesis is usually filled with saline (salt water), so if any leak does occur it will be harmless.

Surgical reconstruction of a missing breast is obviously more involved and requires an especially trained and experienced surgeon. A section of fat with overlying skin based on a small artery and vein to provide its blood supply is transferred to the breast region. In the hands of such a surgeon the resulting appearance,

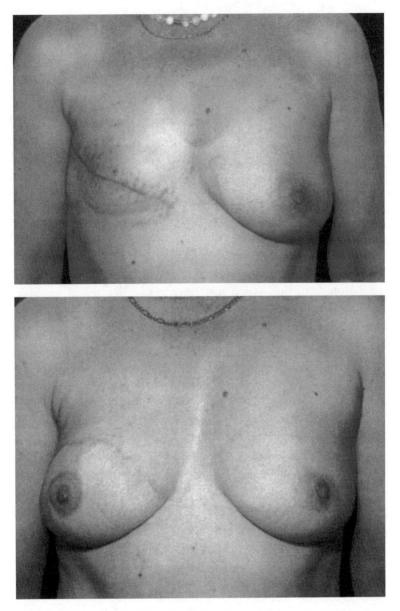

Figure 10.1 (a, above) 'Before' and (b, below) 'after' appearance of a reconstructed breast. Photographs by courtesy of Dr David Pennington (plastic and reconstructive surgeon).

texture, and balance are usually very good. For women who may be a little overweight with a possible roll of fat and flesh to spare in the abdominal area, there may be a further satisfaction in losing some of this fatty tissue to use to reconstruct a new breast. An added refinement of this operation is that in many cases a new nipple can be reconstructed by using nipple-coloured skin, usually available in the labial tissue near the entrance to the vagina (see figure 10.1).

$$\left(11\right)$$

Radiotherapy

Like surgery, radiation therapy can be used in treatment of breast
cancer with the objective of cure. It may also be used to relieve
symptoms (palliation).

External radiotherapy for cure

Two techniques of radiotherapy can be used in treating breast
cancer. The most common, and standard, treatment is with the use
of modern *external irradiation*. Present techniques use linear accelerator high energy irradiation equipment that is available only at
hospitals or institutions with specialised radiation oncology units.
Computerised models assist in planning the best irradiation 'fields';
that is, the size and location of the areas to be covered, the direction of irradiation beams, the doses to be given, and so on.

Simulation procedure for external irradiation

When the patient first attends a radiotherapy department (sometimes if it specialises in cancer treatment it may be called a 'radiation oncology' department) she will be taken to a *simulator room*
for what is called the process of *simulation*. There she will be intro-
duced to technical staff who will take X-rays of the parts of the
body to be treated. They will plan with remarkable precision and
accuracy how much irradiation should be given from different

angles to achieve the greatest effect on the part containing the cancer while causing least damage to surrounding and overlying normal skin and other normal tissues and cells and as little damage as possible to the underlying lungs. Indelible pen marks or little tattoo marks are made in the skin so that for each treatment given on the following days the radiotherapy technician will know exactly where to direct the irradiation.

The whole process of simulation should take no more than one hour and needs to be done only on the first visit. The pinpoint tattoo marks avoid the need to repeat the simulation planning process. Like any other tattoos, these small spots remain in the skin permanently but because they are so small they are not conspicuous and they are not always easy to find.

Delivery of radiotherapy

In most radiotherapy departments the treatment is given only 4 or 5 days in each week. Weekends are free and one day every second week is set aside for servicing the intricate equipment.

In the treatment room the patient will be asked to lie on the treatment couch. Using the skin marks as a guide, the technician will help her get into the best position so that treatment will be delivered in exactly the right direction. The patient is made comfortable and is asked to keep still but to breathe normally.

The radiographer will then go into an adjoining room, which has a glass window so that a close watch can be kept on the patient. An installed microphone system allows the patient and the radiographer to continue to talk to each other. When the treatment equipment is switched on the patient will hear a soft whining noise. The active head of the machine will move around her body, delivering exactly the right amount of irradiation over the right period of time in the right directions to the right parts of the body or 'fields', as previously calculated.

The whole treatment process will take less than half an hour on each treatment day and the actual delivery of irradiation is for only a part of that time.

It is important for the technician giving treatment to stay out of the treatment room while the irradiation is being delivered. Although the dose of irradiation scattered around the room is very small, the technician is doing this work almost every day of his or her working life and the accumulation of even small doses of irradiation would become dangerous.

The precision equipment and computerised designs ensure that the maximum safe and effective doses are given. The objective is for the cancer cells to be repeatedly bombarded so that they accumulate a dose of irradiation from which they cannot recover. This has to be precisely controlled so that any damage to normal tissues or cells is small so they can readily recover from it. The treatment may take 5 or 6 weeks to complete.

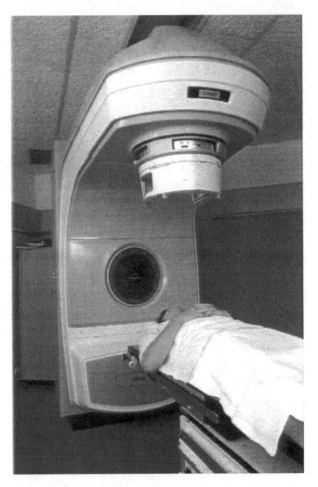

Figure 11.1 This woman is about to begin external radiotherapy.

Brachytherapy

The other radiation therapy technique is called *brachytherapy*. Brachytherapy is not commonly used in treating breast cancer. It is a method of directing radiation right into the cancer itself by inserting wires or tiny pellets ('seeds') containing radioactive materials directly into the cancer. These techniques have been available for some years but not all problems have yet been solved.

The advantage of brachytherapy is that the irradiation is directed precisely into the breast and cancer tissue in greater concentration than is possible with external irradiation, and it poses less risk of damaging the lungs, overlying skin or other nearby tissues. Brachytherapy is therefore usually reserved for treatment of deep-seated cancers or very big cancers. These are cases in which external irradiation may not penetrate sufficiently to affect the whole thickness of the cancer without giving doses of irradiation that would damage overlying skin or underlying lungs. A disadvantage is that without extremely accurate planting of the irradiation materials, some cancer cells may escape the irradiation. Nor will the irradiation field from brachytherapy cover those lymph nodes and other tissues a little distance away from the main cancer mass that might contain some malignant cells. Consequently, brachytherapy is usually given only in conjunction with traditional external radiotherapy. In these cases the external radiotherapy covers the whole area of tissue that might contain cancer cells, and the brachytherapy is given in addition when the main cancer mass is too thick or too deep to be penetrated sufficiently by the external radiotherapy.

There are two main methods of administering brachytherapy. One is by implanting 'seeds' containing a radioactive iodine preparation directly into the cancer region in the breast. These seeds remain in place permanently and emit a measured dose of irradiation directly into the cancer region for as long as the 'seeds' remain radioactive. This is very expensive treatment and the dose of irradiation must be calculated with great accuracy.

In the other form of brachytherapy, radioactive wires are implanted into and through the breast and cancer. These wires are left in place until the measured dose of irradiation required has been completed. If necessary these wires can be adjusted in position. When the required irradiation has been completed the wires are removed. Studies suggest that for some cancers, especially for locally advanced cancers, this treatment probably combined with external radiotherapy may prove to be more effective and also safer than radical surgery.

Adjuvant radiotherapy

Radiotherapy alone is not usually regarded as a method of curing a breast cancer. Alone it is not likely to cure large cancer masses or large lumps of cancer cells. On the other hand, it can often destroy small clusters of cancer cells or individual cancer cells left behind after an operation has removed all visible cancer. When there is some doubt whether all cancer cells have been totally removed during surgery, radiotherapy is often used to destroy any cancer cells that may have been left behind. Radiotherapy used in this way is called *adjuvant* radiotherapy.

Surgery and adjuvant radiotherapy

External adjuvant radiotherapy using a linear accelerator is given as standard treatment to the breast in all those patients where there may be some doubt as to whether all local cancer cells were totally removed. It may be appropriate for patients who have had all or part of a breast containing a cancer removed, and it may be appropriate for some patients who have had total mastectomy possibly with radical surgery but in whom there may have been some doubt as to whether all local cancer cells were totally removed. In such people, surgery followed by radiotherapy should give better chances of cure than surgery alone. However, operation to remove all lymph nodes from the armpit is usually considered safer than radiotherapy of the armpit region. Using both together in the armpit region is best avoided if possible because the radiotherapy can lead later to the development of swelling of the arm or damage to shoulder tissues, resulting in a stiff shoulder.

If there is evidence that the cancer may have spread into lymph nodes in other areas, especially in the lower part of the neck or in the chest, then these lymph node regions should also be irradiated.

Follow-up after radiation therapy

It is important for the doctors to arrange regular follow-up consultations after any form of radiation therapy, especially to determine how effective the radiotherapy has been in treating the cancer. Further treatment possibilities may include need for irradiation to one or two sites of secondaries such as in bone, or need for a more general anti-cancer treatment such as chemotherapy or one of the forms of hormone treatment if cancer could still be present.

Further radiation treatment cannot be given to the breast region as the maximum safe dose would have already been given to these tissues and further irradiation to this region would be dangerous. The past and future doses of irradiation are cumulative, and together more treatment would inevitably risk permanent damage to the lungs and overlying skin and other surrounding tissues.

Radiotherapy before surgery

Cure by surgery alone may not be possible in cases where the cancer has spread throughout the breast or the cancer is a big lump in the breast or it has spread into overlying skin or underlying muscle (stage III breast cancer). In these patients radiotherapy is often used to control the cancer growth, and occasionally radiotherapy might appear to eradicate a large breast cancer totally. In cases where radiotherapy appears to have greatly reduced or even totally eradicated a large cancer in the breast, the surgeon and radiotherapist should then consider together whether it would be advisable for the breast to be removed by operation to reduce the chances of regrowth of cancer in the breast.

Radiotherapy can therefore be used as part of a combined treatment to reduce the size and malignant qualities of the cancer lump, making it smaller so that it may be possible to remove it surgically and give hope of achieving a cure. Such combined integrated treatments are discussed in chapter 13.

Palliative radiotherapy

When there are cancer secondaries in areas of bone or other tissues, radiotherapy can play a very useful role in controlling them. Secondaries in bone causing pain will usually respond to radiotherapy, giving the patient good pain relief. However, there is a limit to how much radiotherapy can be given safely to any patient, so there is a limit to the number of places that can be treated and a limit to the total dose that can be given to any one area.

Side-effects of radiotherapy

During radiotherapy and for some days or even a few weeks afterwards, the patient may feel rather tired and lethargic and possibly depressed. In most people this is a temporary phase that passes without serious incident.

Radiotherapy may cause some minor skin changes like mild sunburn. Breast sensation is often rather different for some time, but this is less noticeable as time passes. Radiotherapy will usually leave some permanent skin redness and possibly increased tightness of underlying tissues. A permanent stiff shoulder or swelling of the arm are not likely if the patient has been encouraged to exercise the shoulder gently after treatment, and especially if radiotherapy and surgery are not both used in the armpit region.

The skin over the irradiated area will sometimes become dry, reddish, itchy and sensitive. Sunbaking or dry heat such as electric blankets will make it worse and should be avoided. Soaps or drying agents like perfumes or some deodorants should be avoided, as should hot baths or hot showers. A moisturising lotion is often helpful. The patient should avoid tight or woollen clothing and should wear loose cotton clothing instead.

The other significant concern is that the underlying lungs cannot be completely protected from irradiation and some patients are left with some degree of lung damage.

(12)

Hormone treatment

The first evidence that breast cancers would respond to hormone treatment was recorded in 1896 at the Glasgow Royal Infirmary and reported in a review by a Scottish doctor, Sir George Beatson. He reported results of studies in that hospital that showed reduction in the size of breast cancers after removal of the ovaries.

Since then it has been observed that removing the ovaries (the main source of female hormones) often resulted in temporary improvement in patients with breast cancer. It has also been known that the male hormones, the androgens, were likely to have a beneficial effect on breast cancers, particularly in younger women.

In the middle of the twentieth century it was common to treat advanced breast cancers with male hormones, or by removing the ovaries, or by removing either the adrenal glands or the pituitary gland. These glands are responsible for hormone production in the body, and advanced breast cancers would often regress, albeit temporarily, after their removal.

Today both hormones and anti-hormones are available. They give similar and better responses without the need to give male hormones or to remove ovaries, adrenal glands or the pituitary gland.

Case report 6 (p.92) is an example of the use of radiotherapy and hormone treatment for an older woman with stage IV breast cancer.

Hormone receptor testing

Breast cancer tissue removed at operation or from a sample taken at biopsy is now routinely tested for sensitivity to certain hormones. These studies are called the oestrogen receptor test and progesterone receptor test. The degree to which these hormones bind to cancer cells indicates whether the cancer is likely to respond to hormone treatment.

Among the longest tried and tested of the presently available products is a drug marketed as *tamoxifen*. Tamoxifen prevents or blocks the action of the woman's own female hormone, oestrogen. In many patients oestrogen is cancer-stimulating. Fortunately tamoxifen is easy to take by mouth and rarely causes unwanted side-effects. However, when it is used for several years there has been a small increased risk of developing cancer in the uterus in some patients. Despite this small risk, it can still be a very useful agent for women to take to control a breast cancer when cure by standard means is uncertain or not possible. Tamoxifen is also sometimes given in a small daily dose as a preventive measure in women who have a high risk of breast cancer. Tamoxifen can reduce the risk for these women of getting a breast cancer.

Trials presently under study suggest that a new anti-cancer drug called *Letrozole* given as an alternative to tamoxifen may be even more effective and appears to pose no greater risk.

A range of other hormone agents is now available and more are under study. They will be recommended by the specialist doctors according to different needs and circumstances.

Case report 6: *Grace, aged 78*

Grace was a 78-year-old widow who complained of severe pain in her right hip as well as some other less severe bone pains. X-rays showed a region of bone destruction in the upper end of her right thigh bone (the femur) as well as some smaller but similar spots in other bones. These looked like areas of probable secondary cancer.

When Grace was examined her doctor found a small hard lump in her right breast and some hard lymph nodes in her right armpit. Grace had not noticed these. The doctor arranged a biopsy, which showed that the breast lump was a cancer. The doctor then arranged bone scans and these showed several small defects that looked like cancer in a number of bones.

Grace was started on tamoxifen treatment and was given one tablet to take morning and evening. She soon got some general pain relief, but X-rays three months later showed that the problem in the hip bone was no smaller. Grace still had hip pain, so treatment of this area of bone with radiotherapy was arranged. This gave her good relief from hip pain for a year, but further pain then developed in the hip and in a number of other bones, and a chest infection also developed. The chest infection was found to be due to secondary cancer in both lungs. Grace was given good palliative care, first at home, then in a nursing home, where she died with widespread cancer a few weeks later.

$$\textbf{13}$$

Chemotherapy

A fourth approach to the treatment of breast cancer is the use of non-hormonal anti-cancer drugs or chemicals. This approach is known as *chemotherapy*.

The first effective anti-cancer chemical agent was discovered more or less accidentally during World War II, but since that time an increasing number of potentially more useful chemical agents with fewer side-effects have become available. There is now a wide range of anti-cancer drugs that damage cancer cells in different ways. Some of these have been found to be effective against most cases of breast cancer, but others are not. Some are effective if used alone, but most are more effective if used in combination with other agents.

The most effective doses, timing and combinations of anti-cancer agents have been found to be different for different cancers. A whole specialist discipline of medical oncology has developed around determining the best use of these agents and hormonal agents, so that a cancer specialist team now consists not only of the family doctor, a surgeon and a radiotherapist but also should include an expert medical oncologist.

Chemotherapy might be used as an adjuvant (or assistant) after surgery to eradicate a small number of scattered cancer cells that may still be present after surgery (see adjuvant chemotherapy, pages 96–7). Sometimes chemotherapy might be used before surgery and/or radiotherapy to make the cancer smaller and so increase the chance that it will be curable by the surgery and/or radiotherapy that is to follow. This is called *induction* or *neoadjuvant* chemotherapy. Another option is to use chemotherapy both before and after surgery, possibly using it and/or radiotherapy in an integrated approach to treating the cancer. Chemotherapy used alone is not often a cure for any cancer, including breast cancer. However, it will often reduce the size and aggressive nature of cancers, including widespread cancers, for some time and might give good relief of symptoms (palliation).

Administration of chemotherapy

There are two main methods of administering chemotherapy. The first and simplest method, and the method most often used, is *systemic chemotherapy*. In this technique, the drugs are usually given into a vein, and the patient's blood circulates them to virtually all parts of the body in more or less equal doses and concentrations.

The other method of administering chemotherapy is called *regional chemotherapy*. It is used only on rare occasions, and then only in highly specialised units, because it is more difficult and more controversial. The drugs are given into an artery that supplies blood to the area containing the cancer, so the chemotherapy is concentrated in the tissue containing the cancer. It can have advantages when the cancer problem is confined to one area or tissue, such as an arm or a leg, and there is one artery that supplies the tissue with blood, but is not often relevant for breast cancer.

Systemic chemotherapy

Anti-cancer drugs are sometimes given by mouth but intravenous injection or intravenous slow infusion over a period (intravenous drip) is more usual.

There are three main objectives of systemic chemotherapy. These are: attempts at achieving a cure; as adjuvant treatment; and to give palliation in the form of long-term control of most of the cancer cells with the aim of giving relief of symptoms.

Attempts at cure

Cure is obviously the most desirable objective for any cancer treatment. There are as yet no anti-cancer agents that are likely to cure
breast cancer by themselves, although on very rare occasions this
happens. Chemotherapy is more likely to be an important part of
achieving a cure when it is integrated with other forms of treatment. Chemotherapy used in combination with either surgery or
radiotherapy or both to treat a big, advanced cancer in a breast has
sometimes achieved a cure when any one of these treatments used
alone would have been unlikely to be successful.

Chemotherapy used first in an integrated program of treatment
is called *induction* or *neoadjuvant* chemotherapy. The objective in
this case is for the chemotherapy to induce changes in the cancer
that make it smaller and less aggressive. This increases the chance
that it will be curable by the surgery or radiotherapy that follows.
In treating a locally advanced stage III cancer in the breast, surgery
alone would be unlikely to eradicate all the cancer. There is the
risk of leaving cancer cells in the operation wound, and these
might then regrow. If the patient is first treated with chemotherapy
the cancer can usually be made to shrink to a smaller size that can
be removed more safely by operation.

Sometimes to be more sure of achieving total eradication of the
whole cancer in the breast, chemotherapy is given first as induction treatment to reduce the size of the cancer, then radiotherapy
is used to reduce it further and destroy more cancer cells. Finally
surgery is carried out to remove the breast containing any remaining cancer cells.

Systemic chemotherapy given in this way circulates to all body
systems, so it may also destroy any cancer cells that might be growing somewhere else in the body. It therefore combines the benefits
of induction and adjuvant chemotherapy. After operation, more
adjuvant chemotherapy is also given intravenously with the objective
of destroying any remaining cancer cells that may still be somewhere else in the body.

Adjuvant chemotherapy

After surgery to cure stage II breast cancer or if surgery has been
carried out to remove a stage III breast cancer, there is always some

concern that the cancer may have already spread into organs or tissues beyond the breast, even though it cannot be detected elsewhere. In these circumstances more patients are cured if systemic chemotherapy is given after the operation as adjuvant chemotherapy.

When the chemotherapy is given intravenously it circulates to all tissues because it is carried in the bloodstream. While the chemotherapy would be unlikely to totally cure any large secondary cancer deposits, in some cases it does appear to eliminate very small hidden clumps of cancer cells wherever they may be. If cancer was found in several of the lymph nodes removed from the armpit, there is a more than 50 per cent chance that there will be some cancer cells somewhere else in the body that cannot be detected by present day methods. If women with these cancers are not given any further treatment, secondary cancer deposits will show up sooner or later in about 60 per cent of cases. However, if these women are given a program of chemotherapy every month for 6 or 12 months after the operation, the risk of cancer secondaries showing up later is reduced by about 12 or 15 per cent. That is, from about a 60 per cent chance of recurrence the risk is reduced to under 50 per cent. The overall length of survival is also increased even in those who eventually do have a recurrence.

Chemotherapy given like this to mop up undetected cancer cells elsewhere in the body is called *adjuvant chemotherapy*. It is usually recommended for women found to have cancer in the lymph nodes, especially if they are reasonably fit and young (usually under 65 or 70 years)—older women do not tolerate the side-effects of chemotherapy as well as younger women. Instead of adjuvant chemotherapy, older women are usually given tamoxifen tablets daily for perhaps two years. Older women are more likely to get benefit from tamoxifen, and it is unlikely to cause troublesome side-effects.

The side-effects of chemotherapy are discussed on pp. 98–9.

Palliative chemotherapy

Chemotherapy is also used in palliation of widespread breast cancer. The cancer may have spread to several places and chemotherapy given systemically will be carried in the blood to wherever secondary cancer growth is present. Widespread breast cancer may be in such places as bones, scattered lymph nodes, skin or fat, other organs like liver, lungs, ovaries or adrenal glands, or even the other breast.

Some breast cancers will respond well to some of the available chemotherapy agents so the symptoms and distress they cause are reduced, but not all respond well. Secondary cancers in some tissues respond better than in some other tissues. There is as yet no reliable way of determining which patients are likely to get good relief other than by trial and error.

In general older patients are more likely to suffer most trouble-some toxicity or side-effects from chemotherapy. For women over the age of 65 or 70 years chemotherapy is not so often recommended, especially without at least trying to achieve a good palliative response with a less toxic hormonal approach, particularly with tamoxifen or a similar anti-hormone medication.

Side-effects of chemotherapy

Unfortunately no matter what anti-cancer drugs are used there is always a risk of toxicity; that is, unwanted side-effects. It is not only cancer cells that are destroyed or damaged by chemotherapy; any growing cell or frequently dividing cell can also be affected by the chemotherapy.

Some types of cell are affected more than others. Hair is constantly growing, so hair-growing cells are often damaged by chemotherapy, resulting in hair loss. The good news is that hair loss and other unwanted side effects are temporary. After completion of treatment the hair grows again, often thicker, curlier, and better than before.

Other tissues commonly damaged by the chemotherapy are bone marrow (resulting in possible temporary anaemia and other effects and requiring regular checking with blood counts), and the lining of the mouth and digestive tract (sometimes causing mouth ulcers or bleeding). A number of other tissues may also be damaged with some drugs, so regular monitoring is required with these drugs. Patients often feel tired, listless and unwell during the course of treatment, but they return to normal after treatment has been completed.

Regional chemotherapy

In some specialised clinics *regional chemotherapy* is used in an attempt to achieve a greater response of an advanced cancer in the breast. The drugs are given directly into specific arteries that supply the breast and the cancer in it with blood. This technique should achieve a greater impact of the drugs because they are able to act in greater concentration directly on the cancer cells before flowing into the general systemic circulation as systemic chemotherapy.

While a number of studies have shown a great impact on the primary breast cancer by this technique, a good and satisfactory initial (or induction) response can usually be achieved by the simpler and more widely available intravenous or systemic administration of the drugs.

Regional chemotherapy for breast cancer is not widely practised. It should certainly be practised only in highly specialised units, as it is controversial whether it has real advantages over systemic chemotherapy and there is potential for additional local side-effects.

Side-effects of regional chemotherapy

Although regional chemotherapy is more likely to achieve a greater impact on the primary cancer in the breast, without skilled and experienced supervision there is a risk that the chemotherapy might not be concentrated in the right place and as a result cause more damage to other tissues than to the cancer. Most successful treatments have been given by continuous flow over five weeks or so with close monitoring and care, and this is very expensive in hospital bed time. An important objection is that for breast cancer it may not be necessary, as good responses can often be achieved by the simpler use of systemic chemotherapy given as induction chemotherapy to reduce the cancer, making it more treatable by follow-up radiotherapy and/or surgery.

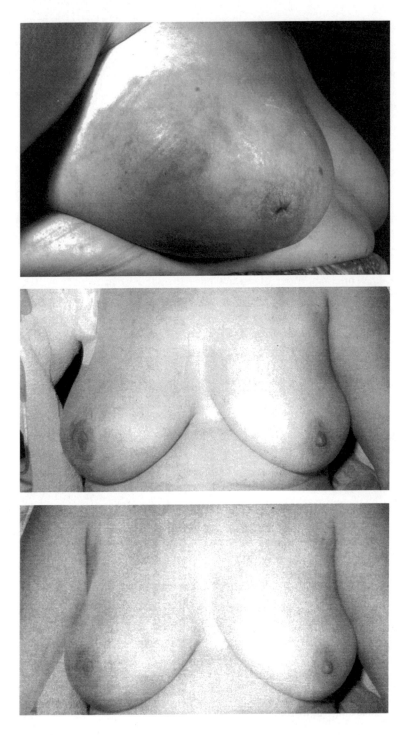

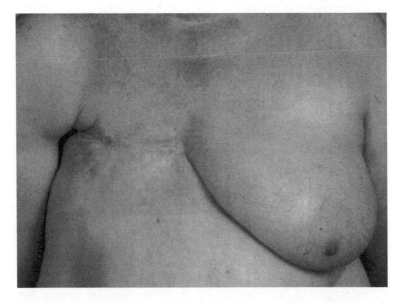

Figure 13.1 Combined integrated treatment in successful management of a patient with an advanced stage III breast cancer. (a, opposite top) The advanced breast cancer when the patient first consulted her doctor. The cancer was involving most of the breast and attached to overlying skin and nipple. (b, opposite centre) After five weeks of continuous induction or neoadjuvant chemotherapy (in this case given by intra-arterial infusion), the cancer had regressed a lot but the breast was still a little enlarged. Radiotherapy was then commenced. The bandages cover the small tube (or cannula) that passes through the skin and into a suitable artery to infuse chemotherapy agents directly into arteries supplying the breast with blood. (c, opposite bottom) Three weeks after completion of a five-week course of radiotherapy. The cancer had further regressed but a reduced firm mass could still be felt in the breast. The patient then had a surgical operation in which the breast and lymph nodes in the armpit were removed. (d, above) The patient was given one year of adjuvant chemotherapy after the operation. This photograph was taken 6 years after surgery and 5 years after adjuvant chemotherapy had been completed. When last seen 14 years after surgery she appeared well and free of cancer.

Case report 7: *Jan, aged 46*

Jan and her husband are farmers with two children. Jan worked hard with her husband on their dairy farm.

Jan gradually became aware that her right breast was enlarging and the overlying skin including the nipple area was a pink colour (figure 13.1a). She consulted her doctor, who arranged mammography and a consultation with a specialist surgeon. The surgeon found a general enlargement and firmness of the right breast, but no enlarged lymph nodes in the armpit. Mammograms showed evidence of a large cancer behind the nipple area in the central region occupying most of the right breast, and biopsy showed cancer cells consistent with an inflammatory breast cancer.

The surgeon suggested to Jan that surgical operation alone was unlikely to be successful in totally removing the cancer, but it was likely that treatment by radiotherapy would control the cancer for a period although cure by radiotherapy alone would also be unlikely. She was advised that hormone treatment should give temporary improvement, but was unlikely to be of long-term benefit. An alternative suggestion was a course of intense chemotherapy, but this would have a risk of side-effects and cure by chemotherapy alone would be unlikely.

The surgeon's next suggestion was that all these treatment approaches could be used in a combined treatment regimen and this might give Jan the best chance of total control of the cancer. However, the surgeon warned that the treatment would be prolonged with possible severe side-effects, and might still fail.

Jan and her husband talked it over with their family doctor and decided they would like to try the combined plan of treatment. This was arranged.

Jan was admitted to hospital, and a suitable program of chemotherapy was planned. As the surgical team had facilities for putting a small tube (a cannula) into the arteries that supplied blood directly to the breast containing the cancer, this was the technique chosen for direct infusion of concentrated chemotherapy to the cancer. Continuous chemotherapy was thus infused into the cancer for five weeks and the cancer gradually became much smaller (figure 13.1b).

Three weeks later a course of radiotherapy to the breast and armpit regions was commenced, and again treatment extended over a period of five weeks. At the end of this time the breast lump was smaller and difficult to feel (figure 13.1c).

Three weeks after the course of radiotherapy was completed, the breast, the overlying skin and the lymph nodes in the armpit were removed at operation.

Three weeks after surgery a one-year course of adjuvant chemotherapy was started.

Although Jan was troubled by nausea, hair loss and other side-effects of treatment for some months, she returned to help her husband on the farm. Fourteen years later she is alive and well and still farming. She has a good head of hair, and there is no evidence of cancer (figure 13.1d).

Case report 7 is an example of effective use of regional chemotherapy in a combined treatment of a woman with a locally advanced breast cancer. It is important to state that although Jan is a real person and her history is as reported, the circumstances of such cases are not common. The medical profession does not know how often such good results can be achieved, and so further research is needed and should be encouraged.

Treatment of breast cancer in men

Cancer of the breast in men is uncommon, but men often wait until a lump under the nipple has been present for a long time before they seek treatment. Fortunately most such lumps in men are benign, but when a cancer is detected it has usually become more advanced and sometimes even ulcerated through the nipple and surrounding skin before the man seeks treatment (see figure 13.2).

Treatment of breast cancer in men is essentially similar to treatment of breast cancer in women, that is, by surgery, radiotherapy, hormone treatment and chemotherapy. Cancers in the male breast often respond to hormone treatment. Removal of the testes (castration) will often be effective for some time in controlling many cases of otherwise incurable male breast cancer, but castration rarely results in complete long-term cure.

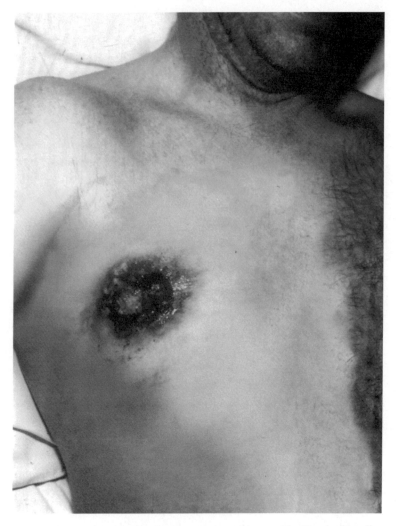

Figure 13.2 Cancer in a breast of a 55-year-old man. The lump under the nipple was already growing through the nipple and surrounding skin when he sought medical advice.

(14)

Follow-up care

Good general health care is important after the initial treatment is completed. The patient should have good nutrition with a good balanced diet, possibly supplemented with adequate vitamins and minerals like calcium taken in tablets or capsules. Regular appropriate daily exercise as well as rest and sleep are important, as is care of any associated problem such as anaemia. Smoking should be avoided.

In spite of good treatment and good follow-up care, difficulties and complications can arise, either from the treatment given or from further disease.

Long-term complications of surgery

Arm pain and paraesthesia

Any extensive operation in the armpit will inevitably damage some of the nerves that pass through the armpit. This may simply leave a numb feeling in the inner region of the upper arm, but occasionally this numb feeling becomes a tingling sensation. Although this sensation, or paraesthesia, does not cause much concern to most patients, some patients find the sensation unpleasant and some may describe it as painful. Most women accept the sensation as being a small price to pay for the hope of being cured of the cancer and do not really notice it after a while, but a small number of patients may need pain-relieving medication or treatment of one sort or another to relieve anxiety.

Lymphoedema (arm swelling)

After a radical mastectomy, which always includes total removal of lymph nodes in the armpit, and particularly if radiotherapy was used in follow-up treatment of the armpit area, swelling (called *lymphoedema*) in the arm is likely. Sometimes there is no noticeable swelling, but in some patients the swelling can be considerable and may impair full use of the arm.

The swelling is caused by interference with drainage of fluid from the arm arising from removal of lymph nodes and surgical and radiation damage to the draining lymph vessels. The arm swelling may be temporary, but it is not uncommon for it to persist for months, years or even permanently. Rest and elevation whenever possible (sometimes with the arm on a pillow when the woman is lying down, or sometimes in a sling when she is up and about), physiotherapy and massage can help in reducing the swelling, but there is no known way of curing severe persistent swelling.

Apart from the discomfort that is often associated with lymphoedema, the tissues in the swollen arm are more susceptible to an infection called *cellulitis*. This may become prolonged, and repeated episodes of cellulitis are common in some women. Care must therefore be taken to protect a swollen arm from damage and risk of infection, and any episode of infection should be treated with rest and elevation of the arm and with early and appropriate administration of antibiotics.

As there is no ready cure for lymphoedema and it can be so troublesome if left uncontrolled, lymphoedema treatment clinics have now been established in many centres to provide good care for women with this potentially disabling problem. In these clinics, especially trained and especially patient and understanding physiotherapists help the patients by using elevation and gravity, massage, pressure bandaging and other techniques to help keep fluid from accumulating in the arm. They also teach their patients how best to care for their swollen arms at home and between visits.

Case report 8 illustrates some troublesome post-treatment complications, including lymphoedema, in a woman treated with chemotherapy, surgery and radiotherapy, and how these problems were managed.

Recurrence of cancer

As for any patient treated for a cancer, there is a constant worry about the possibility that the cancer has not been cured and one day might return, either in the breast or lymph node region or in the other breast or elsewhere. The risk of this happening will depend very much on how early the cancer was detected or how advanced it was before treatment was started. It will also depend on how appropriately it was treated. For these reasons it is imperative that a system of follow-up care be arranged for all patients so that if there is ever any evidence of further trouble it can be attended to without delay.

Most patients with breast cancer can now expect to be cured. This is because good screening methods, self-examination and a general better awareness mean that most women are now diagnosed when their cancer is at an early stage of the disease, and skilled treatment is usually arranged without delay. However cure can never be guaranteed or taken for granted, so regular follow-up examinations are essential. Cancer can recur either locally in the breast or lymph node region or somewhere else in the body. The earlier any recurrence is detected and treated the better is the outlook for the patient.

Pain from secondary (metastatic) sites of breast cancer in bone

One common place for breast cancer to recur is in one or more bones. Recurrence in a bone is usually painful, and the presence of bone metastasis can usually be seen in X-rays or in a bone scan. Sometimes an affected bone will fracture, and this can occasionally be the first indication of a bone secondary (metastasis).

Apart from common pain-relieving medications like aspirin, paracetamol or stronger analgesics, the best treatment of one or two or three bone sites with secondary cancer is usually by radiotherapy to the bone site concerned. Sometimes an orthopaedic surgeon will be needed to pin or plate or otherwise surgically treat any bone that has fractured or is threatening to fracture.

If many bone sites are affected by secondary cancer it may not be practical to give a lot of radiotherapy. For these women, more general treatment, possibly with hormones or chemotherapy, is usually given along with radiotherapy to the most painful sites. If pain control is still not achieved it may be necessary to use stronger analgesics like codeine, pethidine or morphine.

Two new treatments have been developed to give pain relief for people with painful bone secondary cancers. They are *bisphosphonates* and *strontium 89*.

Bisphosphonates

Bisphosphonates are chemical agents that help bones resist destruction by some secondary cancers. They are given by intravenous infusion and become incorporated into the weakened areas of bone, giving some protection and even restoring some of the damaged bone. In doing this they often give considerable pain relief.

For treatment the patient attends a hospital clinic for two or three hours and sits comfortably while a mixture of these agents is given by a slow infusion into a vein. The treatment usually does not bother the patient, but it may need to be repeated at intervals of about one month.

Strontium 89

Strontium 89 is a radioactive element that becomes incorporated in bones and especially in bone tissue destroyed by secondary cancer cells. There it emits a small dose of irradiation, destroying nearby cancer cells. The irradiation penetration is not great enough to penetrate and damage other tissues, except bloodforming cells in the bone marrow. Pain relief is rapid, but because of possible damage to blood-forming cells in bone marrow, especially the platelets responsible for normal blood clotting, the treatment should not be repeated in less than three months and then only if the blood platelet count has returned to normal.

Social, psychological and spiritual help

It is important for cancer patients to have counselling services available to help cope with personal anxieties, family, social and employment anxieties, and other problems that might arise. For some women, a good, patient, and attentive family doctor can be the best person for her counselling needs. Others will be helped by a skilled counsellor, an experienced social worker, a psychologist, or even a psychiatrist with special interest in this field. A member of the clergy can offer some women considerable support and help.

One of the obvious problems for a woman who has had a breast cancer is how best to adjust socially with her family and friends, and especially with her husband or partner. An understanding partner or husband will make her adjustment a great deal more comfortable, especially if the partner attends at least some of the pre- and post-operative medical consultations and counselling sessions. It should not be forgotten that the partner may also need support in meeting changed personal, domestic, social and possibly economic circumstances.

Cancer societies and breast cancer support clubs

Most large centres in Western societies now have organisations whose prime concern is to keep up to date with information and progress so as to allow the best care of patients with cancer. The Australian Cancer Society is one such organisation that is ready to help with advice for care of cancer patients. There are similar organisations in New Zealand, the UK, Ireland, the US, Canada, Japan, South Africa, and all European countries.

Members of breast cancer support clubs predominantly consist of women who have themselves had a breast cancer. They offer great comfort and support for other women with similar problems and anxieties. Breast cancer is now such a common problem for women in Western communities that clubs are now present in most cities and large towns. The experienced friendly support that they offer new members and each other can be invaluable.

On the physical side, help and advice will sometimes be needed in prescribing the most appropriate prosthesis for a mastectomy patient to wear in her bra, or the most appropriate bra for women who have had breast salvage surgery or breast reconstruction. There are a number of manufacturers and retailers of such bras and prostheses who are able to offer helpful advice. The family doctor or the surgeon or people in a breast cancer support club can advise on who best to consult. Experienced nurses in the field can also be of great help, as can other women who have gone through this process themselves.

Palliative care and palliative care treatment teams

When pain cannot be controlled satisfactorily or other problems associated with advanced or widespread cancer cannot be adequately controlled and relieved by the regular treatment team, the help of specialists in palliative care can be invaluable. Practitioners in this specialty include doctors, nurses, dietitians, physiotherapists, sociologists and other experienced helpers. These people are skilled in the best use of medications and procedures for relief of pain and other symptoms. They are also invariably kind, gentle, understanding, and skilled in helping the patient, and in helping her family and other associates and friends who also often need support. Specialist hospices and hospitals are staffed by similarly understanding and skilled people who provide great comfort and help to all concerned—even to members of the regular health-care team.

Case report 8: *Phyllis, aged 67*

Phyllis is the 67-year-old mother of a grown family. She had had a right radical mastectomy operation for breast cancer some seven years previously, followed by rather intense radiotherapy to her armpit region and lower neck because cancer had been found in most of the lymph nodes removed from her armpit.

Phyllis recovered well from the surgery. After surgery and radiotherapy she had been given a course of adjuvant chemotherapy for one year. The chemotherapy had made her feel unwell and she wore a wig for a year to disguise her hair loss, but after the one-year course of chemotherapy was finished she made a good recovery and her hair grew again very well. Her only remaining problem was with poor shoulder movement and some swelling of her right arm. She had difficulty using her right arm for such tasks as hanging out the washing on the clothesline. She had been given physiotherapy for this, and although the movement of her shoulder improved a little the swelling in the arm persisted.

The physiotherapist tried to help by massage from the hand to the shoulder and advised elevation of the arm when Phyllis was in bed. Raising the arm on a pillow was one good way of doing this. The physiotherapist also used compression bandaging to help squeeze fluid from the arm. In spite of this Phyllis had several episodes of increased swelling with redness and infection in the arm, often with a fever. This sometimes followed a minor scratch or other injury to the hand or arm.

Her doctor told her that this condition was called cellulitis, and that 'flare-up' episodes were likely to follow minor injuries or even no injury at all. Apart from taking great care not to injure the arm and to have antibiotic treatment whenever a 'flare-up' occurred, there was no easy cure for the underlying condition. If infection became too frequent the doctor would consider giving Phyllis a small dose of an appropriate antibiotic continuously. The doctor explained that several different types of operation had been tried from time to time to relieve this condition, but that so far none has been satisfactory in the long term. Further studies continue to be carried out in attempts to find a procedure that might be reliable in helping this condition, but as yet a cure has not been found.

Phyllis philosophically accepts that she appears to have had her rather advanced cancer cured and that the arm swelling is a relatively small price to have paid for the cure.

$$\textbf{15}$$

The relationship between the patient and her doctors

Nowhere in the field of medical practice is it more important for the patient to have good personal relationships, trust and understanding than between each patient with cancer and her medical advisers. Breast cancer stands out as having special need for good relationship because of the different possible courses of action that are likely to achieve similar long-term results. The occasion of breaking the bad news to a woman that she has a breast cancer must be handled with gentleness, compassion and understanding. It must not be hurried, and preferably if she wishes it her husband, partner, or a particular friend or family member should be with her. Questions must be answered truthfully and carefully but without unnecessarily stressing pessimistic aspects.

There is no simple answer, and each woman's special needs and priorities and her family and social relationships and circumstances are all important in the decision making.

By the time they reach the age of having need for advice about breast matters, most women will know a family doctor in whom they have trust and confidence. If not they should seek one, perhaps on the recommendation of a friend or friends who have had a similar problem.

After comfortable, unhurried and mutually thoughtful and honest discussion about her problems with her family doctor, and, at least on one occasion, with her husband, partner or other close family member or friend present, arrangements will usually be made for consultation with a specialist.

The specialist is unlikely to be an old family friend, as the family doctor may well be. It is important for the family doctor to arrange referral of the patient to a skilled but compassionate, supportive and understanding specialist who is prepared to listen to the patient's anxieties and take time to answer her many asked or unasked questions. The specialist should be chosen because he or she has special skills, facilities and expertise necessary and is readily available to communicate comfortably with a woman who is probably anxious, worried and confused, and with her anxious, worried and confused family. This is not the occasion for the family doctor to arrange consultation with a specialist because he or she was an old school friend or one who had just come back from overseas with good training and needs support. The relationship between specialist and patient will probably be prolonged over several months or years, and there should be a close three-way relationship with good understanding and communication between specialist, family doctor and patient. Certainly the specialist must have the appropriate skills and facilities and must be up to date with latest information. Over and above this it is most important for the specialist to be able to communicate, explain and be ready to answer questions freely and in an unhurried atmosphere and be readily accessible, possibly by telephone, if or when problems or questions arise.

Discussions about the most appropriate treatment should not sound like an edict from above but must be mutually considered and arranged, having taken into account many factors special to the individual patient. The specialist must also appreciate that no matter how clearly he or she has explained everything to the patient, it is unlikely that the patient will be able to take it all in in one visit. Probably every patient will need one or more further visits, if not to the specialist then at least to the well informed family doctor.

(16)

Uncertainties in medical decision making

It would be good to think that doctors would always know just what was the right thing to do about every health problem in different people under different circumstances. In reality this is not the case. The evidence is not always there for deciding just what is best for each individual patient. Nowhere in the field of medical practice is the situation more uncertain than in some aspects of treating cancer.

Doctors have always had to make decisions and introduce practices and concepts based on the best available evidence. In the past their decisions were usually based on historical evidence or evidence gained by trial and error. Trial and error itself is based on the principle of trying not to repeat mistakes, or of making the least mistakes—this often masquerades as experience.

One way or another, often by making mistakes, new information was produced and progress was made. However much evidence that has been accumulated over many years of medical practice has not been evaluated scientifically and has not been proven to give the best clinical information. Often traditional or historically accepted practices just 'grew' and became accepted without close analysis or criticism. The dominant medical or surgical teacher may have been skilled in practice but unskilled in critical analysis. Each practitioner's own personal experience was often taken as convincing evidence, although it may not have undergone proper analysis or been compared fairly with other evidence or different circumstances. Evidence from a teacher's belief or from personal experience in a limited practice is often referred to as 'anecdotal evidence'. Although anecdotal evidence may well be true, it provides no proof that the outcome seen will be the most consistent if used by different practitioners in different circumstances and for different patients.

There are some notable examples of the value of anecdotal evidence and one-off experiences. Edward Jenner was so convinced that 'vaccination' with the mild disease cow pox would give protection against the deadly and virulent disease smallpox that he tested his belief on himself. He injected himself with cow pox and had a mild reaction. He later injected himself with smallpox and, as he had predicted would be the case, he did not develop smallpox. His belief was based on anecdotal observations and historical evidence. There was no scientifically proven information, yet vital medical progress was made. Edward Jenner's discovery of 1796 has still not been proven scientifically by randomised trials, but the evidence from his one-off experience has provided the basis for eliminating this disease worldwide.

The approach of Edward Jenner in using himself as a test case is still occasionally used in testing strongly held beliefs in other areas of medicine. A report of this type of approach was published in the *Medical Journal of Australia* in 1997 in relation to prostate cancer. A doctor was diagnosed by biopsies as having prostate cancer. Although randomised controlled trials had not been conducted, he believed that there was good evidence that phytoestrogens (plant hormones) could influence the growth of prostate cancer, as do human oestrogens. On this basis he treated himself with a moderate dose of phytoestrogens each day for seven days and then underwent surgery for removal of his prostate gland. The pathologist was asked to compare the appearance of the prostate cancer cells removed at surgery with the appearance of the cancer cells from the biopsies taken before the treatment with phytoestrogens was started. The pathologist found clear evidence of apoptosis (inbuilt cell death) in the cancer after the treatment, although there was no evidence of apoptosis in the biopsy specimens taken three weeks earlier. This one-off study did not prove anything as convincingly as would a scientifically controlled randomised study because it did not show that this treatment would work in other people, but it certainly indicated that there seemed to be a basis for further study.

Evidence-based medicine

Computer technology has made it possible to link new scientifically studied and mathematically confirmed clinical information from randomised studies through a variety of approaches in statistical and mathematical analysis. The information obtained in this way is what is called *evidence-based medicine*, as opposed to information based on one-off experience, a collection of anecdotes, traditionally accepted beliefs, medical folklore, wishful thinking, or folk tales. Information from these other sources may be true, but evidence-based medicine seeks to *prove* that the results are true.

Nowadays most acceptable evidence is based on *randomised trials*. In a randomised trial, a large group of patients with the problem to be researched are invited to take part in a closely watched study. The nature of the trial is explained to them, and if they agree to take part in the study they are allocated into a 'test group'. There are usually two test groups, although in some studies there may be more. The patients are usually divided randomly into the two groups by a lottery-type draw over which the researchers undertaking the studies have no control. Patients in one of the two groups (the 'control' group) are treated by the best known available standard treatment; patients in the other group are treated by the new technique under study. Ideally results are recorded 'blind'; that is, by a third party who does not know which patient was given which treatment. Results of the two groups studied are then compared, usually by an appropriate form of statistical analysis, to discover which was the better form of treatment. Such studies are known as *randomised controlled studies*.

A treatment approach based on a logical hypothesis, but not yet ready for a randomised trial, is sometimes tested in a smaller scientific study called a 'pilot study'. The idea and study proposed are usually put to a group of 'peers' who are well informed colleagues of the researcher for their comment and approval. If the researcher's peers agree that the pilot study seems to be justified, the idea is 'trialled' in a small group of well informed and interested patients who consent to take part. If the initial trial is successful, a further and larger group of patients is studied. In this way new ideas can be tested and new evidence gained under well organised, closely observed and safe conditions.

Shortcomings of evidence-based medicine

Statistically valid evidence-based medicine obtained through well organised randomised trials is the most convincing method of gathering vital information, but it cannot be used to cover all situations and all aspects of medical practice. There are so many variations in disease processes, environmental and social situations, human needs, beliefs, emotions, priorities and interpersonal relationships, as well as medical skills, facilities and practices, that it is not always possible to subject even basic information to scientifically designed statistical analysis.

In some cases anecdotal or historic evidence or information based on a logically proposed hypothesis might still be the best available evidence, and it must still play a part in medical thinking and the gathering of knowledge.

An obvious example of important but uncomplicated information gathered without scientific analysis is that there has never been a randomised study to prove that treating people with pneumonia with antibiotics gives a better outcome than the best non-antibiotic treatment, as used before antibiotics became available. Similarly anecdotal and historic evidence suggests that surgical removal of an acutely inflamed appendix is likely to achieve a better outcome than treatment used in pre-anaesthetic days without the intervention of surgery. But in neither case has a 'controlled randomised study' ever been carried out or analysed statistically. Historical and circumstantial evidence and lots of 'anecdotal' information is there, but a scientifically controlled randomised study has never been analysed. Yet who would doubt the value of treating pneumonia with antibiotics or of surgical removal of an acutely inflamed appendix?

In a more recent context, amputation was the traditional and most effective known treatment for people with advanced cancers in a limb that were too big for successful local surgical removal. Anything less than amputation was known to result in a high risk of the cancer recurring in the same region. Experience in some clinics now indicates that in most cases equally satisfactory results can be achieved by 'shrinking' the cancer with induction chemotherapy first and then using surgery to remove the remaining cancer. This has never been 'proven' in a strictly 'randomised controlled study', and in fact in some clinics amputation is still regarded as the treatment of choice. Ideally the treatment approach should be studied in a properly organised trial, but who would be prepared to ask patients to enter a study in which it depended on the luck of the draw as to whether their limb would be amputated or not? Even if such cooperative patients could be found, would this not be a rather select group of people?

There is the additional shortcoming that not all evidence can be justified by statistics and not all statistics can be justified as evidence. Some relevant information cannot be measured or converted into a computerised model. There is still a need for solutions based on logic and close and personal relationships between medical practitioners and their patients. These relationships and the evidence gained from them must not be lost in the momentum for mathematically based medical science. There is no way to measure such factors as warmth of the relationship and a personal understanding of priorities in social, domestic, spiritual and other circumstances between practitioners and their patients, but they are important in decision making. Just because they cannot be measured it does not mean that they can be ignored or discarded. They do make a difference to outcome as far as people are concerned, and patients are people. Historical evidence, clinical experience, patient belief systems, personal and social priorities and needs and other considerations still must play an important part in clinical decision making. The patient must always be a person first, a person with a health problem, not primarily a health problem to be solved. The relationship between the doctor and patient must be personal and sacrosanct, based on many unmeasurable and intangible aspects of human emotion as well as knowledge, and applied to the immediate health needs as worked out between patient and doctor, not as dictated by 'scientific data' alone.

Evidence and breast cancer

Scientific limitations, variations and uncertainties are very apparent in determining the best treatment for women with breast cancer. Outcomes of investigation and treatment are still unpredictable. Patients' priorities are often quite different. What will be the right decision for one patient will not necessarily be right for another patient. Individual judgment and understanding must play important roles, but these are difficult to measure scientifically. Some years ago, randomised controlled studies on surgical treatment were undertaken in women with breast cancer. These showed that the then standard operation of radical mastectomy with removal of underlying muscles and all nearby lymph nodes from the armpit did not result in any more cures than a 'modified radical' operation in which the breast and lymph nodes are removed but no muscle is removed. It is now known from further randomised trials that, for women with a relatively small cancer in the breast, a breast-saving operation in which only that part of the breast containing the cancer is removed, followed by radiotherapy to the breast, is just as likely to result in cure as the 'modified radical' operation in which the whole breast is removed. Yet some women who have a breast cancer are not comfortable unless the whole breast is removed and they should be entitled to make this decision for themselves if that is their wish. To these women the saving of the breast would be more worry to them than the loss of the breast.

To other women, and especially to many younger women, the breast is emotionally very important. If the whole breast must be removed they would choose to have an immediate operation to reconstruct a breast artificially rather than be left for a period without a breast. Until recently most surgeons were reluctant to reconstruct an artificial breast for at least two years until it was clear that the cancer in the breast region was unlikely to recur. Randomised studies have now shown that this delay does not improve the outlook for the patient, and in most cases she should be allowed to choose immediate reconstruction if she wishes. There are sometimes other variables in patients' wishes that may need to be taken into consideration, such as whether or not to have adjuvant chemotherapy, hormone therapy, radiotherapy or chemotherapy for widespread disease that is not causing symptoms. Some women wish to have their other breast removed, especially if there is a high incidence of breast cancer in their families. This is rarely performed. Most surgeons (including myself) would feel uncomfortable about removing an apparently normal breast. Personally I have never done this, but it must be acknowledged that occasionally it must be considered if, after realistic discussions with more than one member of the treatment team, including a clinical psychologist or psychiatrist, the patient still has a strong wish for it and her anxiety about the risk of a second breast cancer is realistically based. That is, that it is a genuine clinical risk of breast cancer that is being treated and not a psychiatric state of mind for which other operations might be requested at a later date. The ultimate decision on these and other matters must be based on the patient's special and personal priorities and needs as well as on the best evidence available of possible outcomes of different courses of action as known to the doctor and treatment teams and discussed with the patient.

Clinical trials

With so many different ways of treating breast cancers and cancers in general, it is important for major treatment teams to continue to discover which method or methods of treatment are most likely to achieve the best results. As the case reports illustrate, this will depend on many factors, such as the age and place of living and home circumstances of the patient, the degree of advancement of the cancer, which organs are involved, the range of treatments available, any potential side-effects of treatment, and the acceptance by the patient of the treatment options.

In order to compare different treatments in different patients and in different circumstances, it is important for studies to be continued in well conducted clinical trials, as described above. When it is not known which option of treatment is best for patients who have a particular problem, studies are conducted in such trials to compare one treatment option with another. Such studies must be well considered and planned by teams of experts, and must be well conducted in a closely supervised fashion. Usually such trials are best conducted in major teaching hospitals, or at least by expert teams such as those that usually practise in major teaching hospitals. This is the way much progress has been made and will continue to be made in improving treatment for patients with breast cancer, as well as patients with other cancers.

Patients should know that if they are asked to take part in a clinical trial it is not only because the specialists cannot be sure that one treatment to be used is better than the other, but also that in taking part in a study to try to find the answer they will certainly be given closely supervised and highly skilled care. They will also help the experts discover just which treatment achieves the best results. This information will be important for the care of future patients, perhaps including members of their own family or friends, or even possibly for themselves in the future.

$$\left(17\right)$$

Future directions

The future for the cancer sufferer is a mixture of hope and caution. Research continues to make progress in areas of lifestyle and diet, medical screening, diagnosis and treatment, and anti-cancer agents. Naturopathy and practices from different cultures are being examined more seriously by orthodox medicine. However the practice of news media and other organisations to make exaggerated claims of cancer 'breakthroughs' is often an embarrassment to the medical profession and too often causes unnecessary hope followed by disappointment among patients and other interested people. The following comments therefore should be understood to be areas of possible future interest and research without any claim that they will necessarily solve cancer problems. Some possibilities have already proven to be of value, but the extent of the value needs further study. Other possibilities are speculative only and ultimately may not prove to be of any help in cancer care or understanding.

Diet and changes in lifestyle

To avoid cancers in general, people should be encouraged to accept that changes in lifestyle are likely to be needed. Active and passive smoking should be avoided for good health in general, including for reducing the risk of cancer. Other lifestyle changes may also be important, particularly in relation to diet. Especially in

Western countries, people should reduce animal fats in their diets and avoid artificial chemical additives and other contaminants in food. Their diets should include a greater intake of fibre, fresh fruits and vegetables, nuts, grains and protective legumes. Good

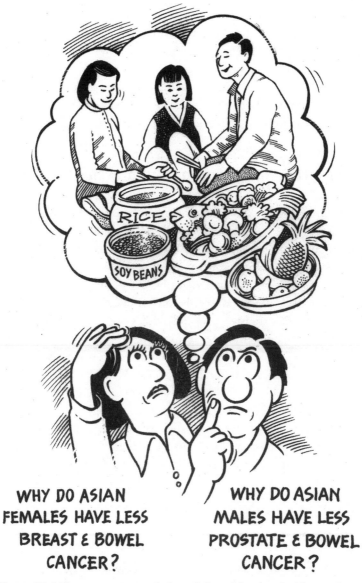

Figure 17.1 The apparent association of diet with a low incidence of certain cancers including breast cancer.

dietary habits should be encouraged from childhood. So should a policy of avoiding sunburn or excessive ultraviolet irradiation, moderation in the use of alcohol, and, especially, not smoking. There will continue to be advances based on clinical and epidemiological information (the study of patterns of disease in the community). These include a further understanding of protective qualities of high fibre diets and the qualities of diets high in other agents that possibly defend against cancer, such as the naturally occurring plant hormones, the phytoestrogens, and the more recently studied extract from tomatoes called lycopene. These particularly apply to the hope of reducing the risk of breast cancer in women, prostate cancer in men, and bowel cancer in both sexes.

Alternative and naturopathic practices

More will be learned from alternative medicine and naturopathic practices as well as from the traditions and practices of ancient and 'undeveloped' communities. However care must be taken to analyse such practices properly and not allow wishful thinking, emotion or fashion to cloud scientific and clinical judgment.

It must be appreciated that, before any new medication can be recommended, extensive tests and studies are necessary to ensure that the agent does not have serious side-effects or toxic properties. Many valuable medicines are extracted from plants, but just because a substance is 'natural' or extracted from plants it does not mean that it is safe to use. Tobacco and betel nut are 'natural' plant products that are known to cause cancer, and the poisons in oleander leaves, rhubarb leaves, apricot seeds, certain mushrooms, and many other toxic and poisonous plants are 'natural' substances. Even strychnine is 'natural', as it is extracted from the seeds of certain plants!

Improved cancer screening

Regular screening of people at special risk for certain types of cancer, and especially breast cancer, is another health measure of increasing importance. This is so that any abnormality that could be cancer may be detected early and treated before a more advanced cancer develops.

It is anticipated that improved, more accurate and simpler screening measures will be available in the future. These may include simple blood tests to screen for cancer antibodies or other so-called 'tumour markers' that may indicate the presence of early cancer before symptoms have developed and when the cancer is at a more curable stage.

Improved early detection, diagnostic and treatment techniques

Further improvements in techniques of detection, diagnosis and management are inevitable.

Improved diagnostic measures will help establish more certain and more accurate diagnosis at an earlier stage. Already improvements in CT scanning and other organ-imaging techniques have made considerable advances in defining the position, extent and tissues involved for some cancers. Magnetic resonance imaging (MRI) has added to these improved diagnostic and imaging methods. It is also anticipated that the new method of organ imaging called PET (positron emission tomography) might possibly make an even greater impact than CT or MRI scanning within a few years because of the additional information it gives about the activity, composition and survival of tumour cells. PET should also help in detection of secondary (metastatic) cancer earlier than has been possible in the past.

Other studies are now being conducted using a newer test called magnetic resonance scanning (MRS). These studies are carried out on breast cancer cells in especially equipped research laboratories, and it is hoped that the results will indicate which anti-cancer agents the cancer cells are most likely to respond to.

The MRS and other new laboratory testing methods will also give information as to which treatment methods and which anti-cancer agents are likely to be of greatest benefit in treating each individual cancer. There will be better methods of screening for and determining more specific anti-cancer treatments for women with breast cancer.

Major progress has already been made in early detection and in establishing the nature of early tumours using fine needle aspiration cytology, core biopsies, frozen section techniques and other improved pathology techniques. The instruments used in these techniques and their application will undoubtedly continue to be improved.

Other potential tests

From time to time potential cancer detection or potential screening tests have been claimed in medical literature and the claims have been repeated in the popular press. These include reports that tests on hair analysis, tests on tears and tests on nipple fluid might all have value in predicting breast cancer. One or more of these and other tests under study may one day prove to be practical and useful in screening for breast cancer, but as yet the only message that can be given with confidence is: 'Watch this space.'

Improved agents and more effective use of chemotherapy

Knowledge is growing about the best use and most appropriate combinations of anti-cancer drugs and most effective treatment schedules. The aim is always to achieve increased anti-tumour activity and reduce the risk of unwanted side-effects. New, more specific and more effective agents, like Letrozole in the hormone group and the taxanes (derived from a plant) in the cytotoxic or chemotherapy group, are constantly adding to the range of available anti-cancer drugs. Other agents that protect bone marrow and other body tissues from harmful side-effects are making the use of many cytotoxic drugs safer and allow more effective doses to be given.

If the ability of bone marrow to produce blood cells has been reduced by chemotherapy, newly discovered *growth factors* can be used to stimulate the bone marrow into producing more blood cells.

Angiostatic and angiotoxic agents

Cancers, like all other tissues, need a blood supply to provide them with nourishment, otherwise they cannot grow or even survive. A new approach in anti-cancer treatment employs agents that damage or destroy the small new blood vessels that grow into a cancer or a metastatic cancer as the cancer develops. Agents have been found that can damage the newly formed fragile blood vessels that supply the cancer with blood, and some of these appear to have potential to destroy or reduce cancers by starving them of blood.

Apoptosis-promoting agents

Another new approach in anti-cancer treatment is the search for agents to promote apoptosis in cancer cells. Normal tissue cells have a limited lifespan. They 'self-destruct' after an apparently inbuilt period of time and are replaced by new cells. This inbuilt self-destructive process is called 'apoptosis'. Cancer cells have lost the ability to self-destruct, but there is some evidence that it may be possible to restore the self-destructive features to at least some types of cancer cells. One of the more interesting studies in this area relates to phytoestrogens or related compounds that seem to have ability to restore some apoptosis properties. This has been shown to be possible in some studies with prostate cancer cells. Breast cancer cells are similarly under study.

Monoclonal antibodies

Greater selectivity in directing anti-cancer agents more directly and in greater concentration to the cancer may be achieved by attaching the agents to *monoclonal antibodies*. Monoclonal antibodies are immune agents that are programmed to attack the cancer cells only. They are programmed to attach themselves directly to the type of cancer cell under treatment. Preparations of monoclonal antibodies are now available for some tumours and treatments based on their use are under study. At the present stage experimental studies give hope that these techniques will be effective and available for clinical use against some cancers, including breast cancer, in the not too distant future. Some interesting results in treatment of breast cancer cells in animal models have been reported but as yet there is no clinical application in treatment of human breast cancer.

Improvements in radiotherapy

Treatment by radiotherapy is also being constantly improved, with different types of radiation emission and different treatment schedules integrated with anti-cancer drugs or hormones. Studies continue, including studies into brachytherapy to administer irradiation directly to the cancer through the implantation of radioactive materials directly into the cancer.

More effective integrated treatments

It does not seem that surgical operations to eradicate cancer will advance greatly over present methods. Organ replacement is not likely to be applicable to breast surgery other than transfer of tissue to reconstruct a breast. Regional tissue chemotherapy infusion techniques (page 99) are one area where advances may still be made.

There is need for an increasing role for better organised and better planned, combined, integrated treatment schedules. In these, chemotherapy, radiotherapy and surgery are used more effectively in combined approaches planned from the outset to improve the treatment of some advanced cancers (see case report 7, page 102).

It is anticipated that in the future, for more cancers that are not already widespread, treatment will be directed more selectively to the affected parts of the body only, possibly as identified by PET scan imaging or by monoclonal antibodies. The treatment will be selectively concentrated where it is needed. This will be an improvement on the present common practice of giving chemotherapy into the general bloodstream so that it is carried in more or less the same dose and concentration to all parts of the body, cancerous and non-cancerous tissues equally.

Bone marrow transplantation

Bone marrow transplants have been tried in another approach in treating patients with widespread breast cancer. Bone marrow transplants have been used successfully in recent years in treating some people, especially children, with leukaemias or lymphomas. In this approach, cancer cells are killed with extremely large and toxic doses of chemotherapy. This also kills blood-forming cells in the bone marrow, but the patient's life is rescued by protective bone marrow transplantation. Some trials have now been reported using a similar approach to treat women with widespread breast cancer. However there are still a number of difficulties and problems to be solved before this approach can be usefully applied. The technique is difficult and expensive and poses special risks, and so far results have been no better than those achieved with standard chemotherapy treatments.

Heat therapy

It is known that cancer cells are more sensitive to heat damage than are normal cells. Studies of the application of heat to eradicate tumour cells selectively, possibly in combination with anti-cancer drugs, may produce improved treatment techniques for certain types of cancer in the future. As yet there is no evidence that this will apply to breast cancer in the immediate future.

It may prove possible to apply heat in using regional chemotherapy and/or regional immunotherapy. Localised heat might well make chemotherapy or immunotherapy more effective in the region heated. A technique called closed-circuit perfusion uses a pump to circulate fluid through the blood supply in one organ or one part of the body. It is kept separate from the normal blood supply to the rest of the body, and can be used to circulate and recirculate anti-cancer agents at relatively high concentration.

Some other advanced localised cancers treated with closed circuit perfusion chemotherapy have been found to be more responsive when the anti-cancer agents are perfused in greater concentration and in a heated perfusion circuit. Such techniques may be applicable to some metastatic breast cancers, for example metastases in the liver, but it is unlikely they will readily apply to treatment of a primary breast cancer.

Cryosurgery

Extreme cold by freezing is also used to treat some cancers. For some years it has been a common practice to treat some small skin cancers by freezing them with a liquid nitrogen spray. Freezing with subsequent thawing destroys cells, including cancer cells. At present a development of these cryosurgery techniques is sometimes used in treating cancers in the liver, and it has now been used with success in some clinics in treating some cases of secondary breast cancer in the liver. However it appears unlikely that there will be any immediate application of this treatment to primary breast cancer.

Electrolysis

Electrolysis is another approach to destroying cancer cells, using probes inserted into the tumour region. At this stage the technique is being studied for its potential in destroying cancer masses in the liver, but any immediate application to treatment of primary cancer in the breast appears unlikely.

Immunotherapy

A long anticipated hope for the future in cancer treatment in general lies in the field of immunotherapy. Cancers are often thought to be due to a deficiency in the body's immune defence system. Whereas abnormal cells are usually recognised and eradicated by the body's natural immune defences, in the cancer patient the abnormal cells have continued to survive and multiply. There is a great deal of supportive evidence for this 'immune surveillance theory', but one piece of evidence lies in the fact that very occasionally a really advanced and aggressive type of cancer will suddenly and spontaneously disappear without trace for no apparent reason. This suggests that somehow the body's natural defence mechanisms have taken charge again.

A great deal of work has been carried out in leading hospitals, cancer institutes and other institutions in the search for greater knowledge and application of the immunological defence mechanisms. Specific immunological tumour markers may reveal evidence of the presence of certain cancers very early, before they can otherwise be detected clinically. Tumour antibodies may not only reveal early evidence of cancer but monoclonal antibodies may be used in treatment, either in a direct attack upon cancer cells or by carrying cytotoxic chemical agents specifically to the cancer cells. There is hope that a more reliable means of stimulating the immune defence system to eradicate cancer cells will emerge from these studies.

Studies with other products of the immune defence system, such as interferon and the interleukins, have not yet had the impact originally expected. However a more recent product, tumour necrosis factor (TNF), may have more immediate practical value, especially when used in combination with other anti-cancer agents in localised intra-arterial regional chemotherapy programs.

Genetic engineering

New techniques of molecular DNA biology offer a different approach in combating cancer. It may soon be possible to change genes in cells that control cell division and cell death. By this means it may be possible to change actually or potentially malignant cells into cells without the tendency to malignant growth. The new science of genetic engineering also has potential for changing the basic nature of cells to prevent cancer developing, or possibly even to change the nature of cells already showing malignant features. Although there have been some small trials of gene therapy, unfortunately there is as yet no evidence that application of these techniques will solve present problems of breast cancer.

Prevention of metastases

A great deal of interest and hope has been created by recent reports that chemical agents called bisphosphonates appear to protect against the development of bone metastases (secondary bone cancers). It may be that these substances have ability to promote apoptosis (self-destruction) in the cells forming metastases in bone.

Improved palliative care

For those people with advanced cancer who are experiencing great discomfort or pain, methods of relieving the suffering with understanding counsel and comfort are now better understood. Such measures are now more readily available, and there is little need for patients to suffer greatly from pain or other distressing symptoms of cancer. Palliative care specialist units are constantly improving care and relieving distress of patients with cancer, including patients with advanced breast cancer.

18

Conclusion—even more hope

As for any health problem, and especially cancer, the greatest hope for the future is in its prevention. *The best cancer treatment is to do everything you can not to get one.*

Although breast cancer has become the most common cancer other than skin cancer affecting women in Western societies, it does appear that it may now have reached or even passed its peak incidence. In the US, lung cancer is now threatening to become more common than breast cancer, but breast cancer is still very common in women. About 1 in 12 women may expect to encounter breast cancer in their average life span of between 75 and 80 years. More is now known about preventable factors or at least factors that should help to lower the risk of breast cancer. Acting on these should help reverse the past trend of increasing incidence. Self-examination and screening for cancer in women at risk and general awareness of the problem among women and members of the medical, nursing and other health professions have resulted in many more breast cancers being detected and treated at an early and curable stage. Increasing numbers of women are now being cured and there are continuing improvements in overall results, including cosmetic results.

With increasing information and comparison of women and communities with high and low incidence of this cancer, there are now encouraging prospects of reducing the incidence of breast cancer in women of Western communities. The best practical prospects for this appear to lie in either significant dietary changes or in adding missing ingredients to traditional Western diets. An acceptable solution for most Westerners could be simply to reduce the content of animal fat in their diets and include more plant food, and in addition to take a daily tablet containing the most likely missing protective ingredients (see pages 20–2 and 34–6).

Screening of women at risk has improved the outlook for women with breast cancer at its earliest and most curable stage. The value of these screening techniques is becoming more widely recognised and screening clinics are becoming more widely available. The rise in breast cancer deaths seen in the twentieth century appears to have passed its peak and the incidence now appears to be on the decline.

In the past, standard surgical treatment in most cases included removal of the whole breast. Nowadays in 80 per cent of cases, treatment without removal of the whole breast can be offered with equally good long-term results. Even if the breast is totally removed, the breast can be reconstructed with good appearance in the majority of women.

For women with serious but not terminal disease, hope must be maintained. The probability or possibility of cure is now available for increasing numbers of patients with cancer. It is important to remember that most women with breast cancer will be cured. However, even for patients for whom prospects of complete cure are not good, worthwhile tumour control and palliation is now available. There is the hope that, for some, further improvement in treatment methods, even prospects of cure, may be around the corner. Results are improving and will continue to improve.

Attention to prevention, early detection and improved treatment methods all depend on constant awareness and vigilance of women and medical practitioners. The need for continued studies and research, including clinical trials, is also apparent. Well conducted research has achieved, and will continue to achieve, constant improvements and is worthy of support from us all. Research teams are constantly making progress, and well conducted research must be supported. Not every research project will be a winner, but some will make new and important discoveries.

Glossary

acute

Sudden; having a sudden, severe and short course.

adenoma

A benign (not malignant or cancerous) tumour in which the cells are derived from glands or from glandular tissues such as the glandular secreting cells in the breast or the lining of the stomach.

anaemia

A blood condition with reduced numbers of red blood cells and/or in which the amount of haemoglobin is reduced.

anaplasia, anaplastic

More extreme abnormality of cancer cells. Breast cancer cells are described as anaplastic when they have lost the special and distinctive features of breast cells. Anaplastic cells tend to be more aggressively malignant. They more readily invade surrounding tissues and spread more readily to other places to grow as secondary cancers (metastases).

angiostatic and angiotoxic

Every cancer and every cancer secondary tumour must have a blood supply to survive. Without a blood supply the cancer cells will die. All cancers therefore develop small new blood vessels (capillaries). A new approach in cancer research is to find drugs or other ways of stopping new capillaries from developing in the cancer and 'feeding' the cancer. The process of stopping new capillaries from developing is described as angiostatic and the process of destroying new capillaries that have developed is described as angiotoxic.

antibody

A type of protein produced by the immune system that recognises invading germs or other substances as foreign. The antibody attaches itself to the invading substance to try to destroy it.

apoptosis

An inbuilt ability of cells to undergo self-destruction after they have served their function. Part of the ageing process of replacement and turnover of ageing cells during normal life. Cancer cells seem to have lost this inbuilt self-limiting life process.

aspiration

Act of sucking up or sucking in or sucking out.

atrophy

Wasting away. Losing special qualities (verb or noun).

axilla

The armpit.

axillary node sampling

Removing a sample of lymph nodes from the armpit for biopsy.

benign

Not malignant. Favourable for recovery. Unlikely to be dangerous.

benign mammary dysplasia

An abnormal development of cells in breast tissue. Although they are abnormal, the cells are not malignant (they are not cancerous). They might develop cysts or solid lumps of glandular or fibrous cells. Sometimes called fibrocystic disease, fibroadenosis cystica, hormonal mastopathy or 'chronic mastitis'.

biopsy

A small sample of tissue taken to be examined under a microscope.

bisphosphonates

Chemical substances that can help bones resist destruction by metastatic (secondary) breast cancer. The bisphosphonates become incorporated in the weakened areas of bone, restoring some strength to the bone and giving the bone some resistance to further destruction.

blue dye test

Injection of a blue dye into the breast near the cancer site; within a few hours the dye will collect in the sentinel nodes, identifying them so they can be removed for biopsy.

brachytherapy

A method of applying radiotherapy by placement of tiny radioactive pellets (seeds) or wires directly into a tumour.

breast-conservation (breast-saving) surgery
> An operation on the breast in which the whole breast is not removed so that the breast can be left to look as normal as possible.

cancer
> A malignant growth of cells. A continuous, purposeless, unwanted, uncontrolled and destructive growth of cells.

capsule
> The fibrous membrane covering that encloses a tissue or organ.

carcinogen
> A substance that causes cancer.

carcinoma
> A cancer of gland cells or cells lining a hollow organ or duct or cells of skin or other body surface. Carcinomas are the most common form of cancer.

CAT scan
> See CT scan.

cell
> The structural living unit of which all tissues and organs are composed.

cellulitis
> A chronic infection of soft tissues with occasional flare-ups. It can occur in the arm after removal of lymph nodes in the armpit interferes with the drainage of lymphatic fluid from the arm.

chemotherapy
> Treatment with chemical agents or drugs.

chronic
> Persisting for a long time. Having a long or protracted course.

chronic mastitis
> A long-standing inflammation or long-standing infection in a breast is accurately described as chronic mastitis. However, the gradual degenerative changes in the condition now called by many names, including benign mammary dysplasia, cystic fibrosis and fibrocystic disease, are often referred to as 'chronic mastitis'.

closed-circuit perfusion
> In cancer treatment, perfusion or closed-circuit perfusion are terms used to describe the use of a pump to provide circulation of fluid through an organ or tissue such as the liver or a limb. The pump system is isolated from the normal body circulation so that the pump pumps the blood or other fluid through that part of the body only, quite separated from the normal blood circulation of the heart and lungs.

congenital

Present from the time of birth.

core biopsy

A special technique of taking a biopsy sample of a tissue by inserting a special needle thick enough to include a sample of the tissue in the needle. The instrument has a cutting edge that allows a piece of the tissue to be included in its hollow barrel part so it can be removed for microscopic study.

CT scan (CAT scan or computerised axial tomography)

A method of visualising body tissues by using special computerised radiographic techniques. These give X-ray pictures of sections of body tissues.

cyst

A fluid-filled sac.

cytotoxic

Having a toxic or harmful effect upon cells. Usually used to describe drugs that have an especially toxic effect on cancer cells.

DNA

Deoxyribonucleic acid; the material from which the body-building genes and chromosomes are made.

dysplasia

An abnormal development of cells in a tissue. Although abnormal, the cells are not malignant (not cancerous).

epidemiology

The branch of medicine dealing with the distribution of disease in the community and causes and spread of diseases.

epidemiological

To do with epidemiology.

fat necrosis

A benign hard lump that can form following damage to fat cells or fatty tissues.

fibroadenosis cystica

This was a common name for the benign breast condition now often called fibrocystic disease or benign mammary dysplasia. It is a good and very descriptive name as the condition is benign and often develops cysts and fibrous or glandular lumps.

fibrocystic disease

A common but benign condition of breast tissue in which lumps form. These consist of cysts and lumps of fibrous or gland tissues. It seems to develop over the years of menstrual activity due to a minor imbalance of hormones. It has been called by many names, including 'chronic mastitis', fibroadenosis cystica, hormonal mastopathy and benign mammary dysplasia.

fibroma

A benign (non-cancerous) tumour composed of fibrous tissues and the cells that form fibrous tissue.

frozen section

A technique for preparing a small sample of tissue for immediate microscopic examination. For normal standard pathology, the tissue specimens are prepared in wax blocks in a process that takes several days. This allows very thin slices of tissue to be cut. The thin tissue slices are then stained and examined. Frozen-section examination allows the tissue specimen to be made hard in a few minutes by freezing it. Freezing makes it hard enough to be sliced thinly immediately. The thin specimens can then be stained and examined under a microscope straight away. An answer can usually be given in a matter of minutes as to whether cancer cells are present.

gene

One of the units that make up a chromosome inherited from parents. Each gene is responsible for a different cell function or inherited characteristic. Genes are located in chromosomes, and chromosomes are composed of the DNA material in the nucleus of cells.

genetic

Inherited. A feature inherited through a gene that was passed on by a parent.

gland

A tissue or organ that manufactures and secretes chemical substances necessary for maintenance of normal health and body function.

hormone

An active biological chemical that is secreted into the bloodstream by glands or organs and which has an effect on the structure or function of other tissues or organs.

hormonal mastopathy

Another name for benign mammary dysplasia, fibrocystic disease or fibroadenosis cystica. As the name suggests, the condition is related to hormonal activity.

hyperplasia

Enlargement of a tissue or organ. Not a tumour but enlargement due to increased numbers of cells. A benign enlargement.

immunotherapy
Treatment of disease by giving immune substances or by stimulating the immune system of body defences.

induction
The process of starting a change or starting something to happen.

induction chemotherapy
The use of chemotherapy to begin changes in a cancer as the first step in an integrated cancer treatment program. The cancer is usually made smaller and less aggressive by the use of induction chemotherapy, which it is hoped will make it more curable by following treatment, usually surgery or radiotherapy or both.

infiltrating or **invasive**
When used in reference to cancer, these terms are used to describe cancers with cells that gradually permeate or creep into surrounding tissues.

infusion
In cancer treatment, infusion describes the method of adding a constant flow of another fluid to the circulation of blood. Often a type of pump is used.

in situ
When used in reference to cancer, this term means the cancer cells have not spread into adjacent or surrounding tissues. Non-infiltrating; the opposite of infiltrating.

ionising radiation (**ionising irradiation**)
Radiation capable of passing through tissues and tearing apart the genetic material in a cell. Cancer cells are generally more easily damaged by irradiation than are normal cells.

isoflavones
A class of plant hormones (phytoestrogens) that are present in many plants but especially plentiful in legume plants like the soya bean. The greatest known source is the red clover plant, a legume that contains all the phytoestrogens found to be most active in human physiology.

isotope
Many elements can occur in different forms or isotopes. Some of these forms are radioactive. Minute amounts of radioactive isotopes known to concentrate in certain tissues are used in medicine to allow scans to detect the presence or absence of these tissues in different normal or abnormal parts of the body. For example certain radioactive isotopes

can be used to allow scans to detect the likely presence or absence of cancer cells in bones.

legumes

A class of plant that includes members of the bean and pea families. All plants of this type contain relatively large amounts of the isoflavonoid phytoestrogens.

Letrozole

One of the more recent anti-cancer drugs presently under study and one that shows encouraging potential in treating advanced cancers.

leucocyte

The 'white' or colourless type of cell that circulates in the blood and is chiefly concerned with defending the body against invasion by foreign organisms or bacteria.

liver

The largest solid organ in the body. It lies in the upper abdomen predominantly on the right side and under cover of the lower right ribs.

lumpectomy

Surgical removal of a lump.

lycopene

The natural red colouring matter in certain plants and especially in tomatoes. It is an anti-oxidant that appears to prevent growth of some cancer cells in culture, including breast and prostate cancer cell cultures.

lymph glands

See lymph nodes. Although commonly called glands, these little structures are not glands and are more correctly called lymph nodes.

lymphocyte

One of the types of white cells that circulate in the blood and take part in immune reactions and the body's defence reactions. A type of white blood cell produced by lymph nodes and other lymphoid tissue.

lymphoedema

Persistent swelling in a tissue as a result of tissue fluid accumulating in the tissues. Lymphoedema in an arm may follow removal of or radiotherapy to the lymph nodes in the armpit because of damage to the draining lymph vessels. It is most likely to occur if both surgery and radiotherapy have been used in the armpit.

lymphoid tissue

A tissue that is mainly composed of lymphocytes and lymphocyte-forming cells and which therefore is part of the body's defence system.

For example, tonsils and adenoids and lymph nodes are composed predominantly of lymphoid tissue.

lymphoma

A neoplastic disease or cancer of lymphoid tissue.

lymph nodes

Small bean-shaped masses or nodules of lymphoid tissue normally 1 to 25 mm in diameter. They are scattered along the course of lymph vessels and often grouped in clusters. They form an important part of the body's defence system. They function as factories for the development of lymphocytes and filter bacteria and foreign debris from tissue fluid. They are not glands but are commonly referred to as 'lymph glands'. There are clusters of lymph nodes in the armpits.

lymphoscintigraphy

The injection of a weakly radioactive tracer substance into the breast near a cancer; the tracer collects in the sentinel nodes so they can be identified for removal and biopsy.

lymph vessels or **lymphatics**

The small vessels that drain tissue fluid into lymph nodes and interconnect groups of lymph nodes. Eventually the larger lymph vessels drain this fluid into the bloodstream. Lymph vessels are rather like fine colourless veins in the tissues.

malaise

A general feeling of tiredness, lack of energy, and ill-health. Feeling unwell.

malignant

Life-threatening. A condition that in the natural course of events would become progressively worse, resulting in death. A malignant growth or cancer is a growth of unwanted cells that tends to continue growing and to invade and destroy surrounding tissues. It also tends to spread to other parts of the body, causing destruction of other tissues.

mammogram

Special X-rays of the breast in which very small doses of X-rays are used to show tissues of different densities in the breasts.

mastectomy

Surgery to remove the breast.

metastasis

Metastatic cancer is a secondary growth of malignant cells that has spread from a primary cancer in another part of the body. Sometimes called a secondary or secondary cancer.

MRI

Magnetic resonance imaging. A technique that allows pictures similar to CT scans to be taken of cross-sections of the body, head or limbs.

mutation

A change or alteration. Sometimes a gene may change so that the offspring may develop certain characteristics not present in either parent. The resulting *mutant gene* may introduce a different structure or function to the growing tissue. Mutation of a gene can occasionally be caused by irradiation or certain chemicals, but most often the cause of mutation is not known.

neoplasm

New growth. An abnormal growth of body cells. A neoplasm may be benign (non-cancerous and usually harmless) with limited growth, or malignant (cancer) with continuous, unwanted, unlimited and uncontrolled growth.

oncogene

An abnormal form of a gene that is responsible for cell division and tissue growth or repair.

oncology

The study of tumours or the study and care of patients suffering from tumours.

Paget's disease of the nipple

A feature of one type of breast cancer in which a crust or small rash appears on the nipple.

palliative

Giving relief (palliation); relieving symptoms but not curing the condition.

PET scan

Positron emission tomography. A technique that gives pictures of body tissues based on different levels of biochemical activity in the tissues.

phytoestrogens

Naturally occurring oestrogen-like hormones present in all plants but in large quantities in certain leguminous plants such as soya beans. Phytoestrogens are thought to be at least partly responsible for the lower incidence of some diseases (especially of breast and prostate) in people (such as Asians) who have a high intake of legumes in their diets.

platelets

Small disc-shaped particles in the blood that are essential for blood clotting.

polyp

A tumour projecting on a stalk from the mucous membrane lining the cavity of a hollow organ.

pre-invasive

In reference to cancer, a cancer that has not yet begun to infiltrate or spread into surrounding tissues. An 'in situ' cancer.

primary or **primary cancer**

A cancer at the place where it started to grow. A primary cancer of the breast refers to the cancer where it started in the breast and not to a metastasis or secondary spread in another part of the body.

prosthesis

An artificial replacement for a missing part.

prosthetic

To do with a prosthesis.

proto-oncogene

A gene that is responsible for cell division and if changed may become an oncogene that can be responsible for a cancer.

radical

Extreme. A radical mastectomy is removal of the whole breast together with nearby lymph nodes in the armpit. Sometimes muscle under the breast is also removed.

radio-opaque material

A substance that does not allow penetration of X-rays. It thus shows as white area on an X-ray film. It is commonly referred to as 'dye'.

radiotherapy

Treatment with X-rays or gamma rays.

red clover

A type of clover plant. A legume that contains the highest known concentration of the isoflavonoid phytoestrogens.

retention cyst

A cyst formed by blockage of a duct such as a milk duct.

sarcoma

A cancer of connective tissues such as muscle, fat, fibrous tissues or bone.

screening test

A relatively simple, safe, reliable and easily performed test that can be carried out on large numbers of people to determine whether they are likely to have a cancer or other serious disease.

secondary or **secondary cancer**

A cancer metastasis. A cancer that has spread from its 'primary' or site of origin and is growing in another tissue or organ.

segmentectomy

In relation to breast cancer, removal of that section or segment of the breast that contains the cancer.

sentinel node

A lymph node into which lymph vessels from a tissue first drain. It is therefore the lymph node most likely to be affected by a spreading cancer.

sentinel node sampling

Removal of sentinel nodes for biopsy to check for cancer spread.

side-effect

An effect other than the effect wanted.

soft tissues

Tissues like fat, muscle, fibrous tissue, nerves and blood vessels between the skin and underlying bone.

soy

An extract of the soya bean, rich in phytoestrogens.

soya bean

A commonly eaten bean, rich in protein and carbohydrate and which contains relatively large quantities of the isoflavones or isoflavonoid phytoestrogens. Soya beans are easily grown and cheaply produced legumes and form an important part of the staple diets of most Asian communities.

spleen

A solid organ containing many blood vessels, located in the upper left abdomen under the protection of the lower left ribs. Its main function is to filter the bloodstream of old or damaged blood cells.

strontium 89

A radioactive isotope of the metal strontium. Like calcium, strontium accumulates in bone, especially in active areas of bone where cancer cells are growing. The radioactivity of strontium 89 (beta irradiation) destroys nearby cancer cells but does not penetrate into other tissues to cause damage elsewhere.

tissue

A layer or group of cells of particular types that together perform a special function.

toxic

Poisonous.

trauma

Injury.

tumour or **tumor**

A swelling. Commonly used to describe a swelling caused by a growth of cells, a new growth or neoplasm that may (or may not) be a cancer. 'Tumor' is the American spelling.

ultrasound scan

A type of scan that uses echoes of very high frequency and hence inaudible sound waves to form an image. It is useful for studying soft tissues and hollow organs that do not show up on X-rays, and is much cheaper and simpler to perform than tests such as MRI. It is also completely safe to use, even during pregnancy.

Further reading

Bishop, J. 1999, *Cancer Facts*, Harwood Academic Publishers, Amsterdam.

Dixon, M. & Sainsbury, R. 1993, *Diseases of the Breast*, Churchill Livingstone, London.

Herman, C., Aldercruetz, T., Goldin, B. R. et al. 1995, 'Soybean phytoestrogen intake and cancer risk', *American Institute of Nutrition*, 757S–770S.

Liew, L. 1999, *The Natural Estrogen Book*, Group West Publishers, Berkeley, California.

Rees, G. J. G., Goodman, S. E. & Bullimore, J. A. 1993, *Cancer in Practice*, Butterworth–Heinemann, Oxford.

Scott, R. 1981, *Cancer—the Facts*, Oxford University Press, Oxford.

Stephens, F. O. 1988, 'Why use regional chemotherapy? Principles and pharmacokinetics', *Regional Cancer Treatment* 1: 4–10.

Stephens, F. O. 1995, 'Induction (neoadjuvant) chemotherapy: Systemic and arterial delivery techniques and their clinical applications', *Australian & New Zealand Journal of Surgery*, 65: 699–707.

Stephens, F. O. 1997, 'Breast cancer: Aetiological factors and associations', *Australian & New Zealand Journal of Surgery*, 67: 755–60.

Stephens, F. O. 1997, *Cancer Explained*, Wakefield Press, Adelaide.

Wragg, M. 1998, *The Cancer Prevention Diet*, Pan Macmillan, Sydney.

For information on breast reconstruction: Australian Society of Plastic Surgeons' website www.asps.asn.au

Index